T0144632

BASIC HEALTH
PUBLICATIONS
USER'S GUIDE

TO
GINKGO
BILOBA

Learn What You Need
to Know about What
Ginkgo Biloba Can
Do for Your Heart
and Mind.

HYLA CASS, M.D.
& JIM ENGLISH
JACK CHALLEM Series Editor

The information contained in this book is based upon the research and personal and professional experiences of the authors. It is not intended as a substitute for consulting with your physician or other healthcare provider. Any attempt to diagnose and treat an illness should be done under the direction of a healthcare professional.

The publisher does not advocate the use of any particular healthcare protocol but believes the information in this book should be available to the public. The publisher and authors are not responsible for any adverse effects or consequences resulting from the use of the suggestions, preparations, or procedures discussed in this book. Should the reader have any questions concerning the appropriateness of any procedures or preparation mentioned, the authors and the publisher strongly suggest consulting a professional healthcare advisor.

Series Editor: Jack Challem
Editor: Roberta W. Waddell
Typesetter: Gary A. Rosenberg
Series Cover Designer: Mike Stromberg

Basic Health Publications User's Guides are published by Basic Health Publications, Inc.

Copyright © 2002 by Hyla Cass and Jim English

ISBN: 978-1-59120-019-2 (Pbk.)
ISBN: 978-1-68162-854-7 (Hardcover)

CONTENTS

Introduction, 1

1. Discovery of a Living Fossil, 5

2. Ginkgo Biloba and the Brain, 15

3. Ginkgo and the Heart, 23

4. Ginkgo and Sexual Enjoyment, 33

5. Ginkgo and Vision, 41

6. Ginkgo and Hearing Disorders, 53

7. Ginkgo's Other Health Benefits, 59

8. How to Select and Use Ginkgo, 65

9. Ginkgo Safety and Cautions, 73

Conclusion, 77

Selected References, 79

Other Books and Resources, 85

Index, 87

INTRODUCTION

Ginkgo biloba is the best-selling prescription herb in Europe, the fifth most widely used herb in the United States, and one of the most highly sought-after herbs in the world, all for good reason. It became one of the most highly prized natural supplements because of its proven effectiveness for enhancing memory and mental function, improving blood circulation to the brain, reducing inflammation, relieving allergies and asthma, and protecting the body from the effects of aging. Ginkgo's well-earned reputation is supported by more than thirty years of scientific and clinical research. In this book, we are going to outline a number of these studies and let you see for yourself the important benefits this magnificent herb has to offer.

A major health threat facing humans, especially aging baby boomers now entering middle age, is the decline in their mental abilities. The decline was traditionally accepted as a normal part of the human aging process, but that idea is now being discarded as an outmoded concept, and treatment for this formerly accepted process is now regularly sought out. The result is that healthcare providers and medical professionals are struggling to cope with the growing flood of older people and their caregivers all looking for ways to treat dementia, memory impairment, and other age-related cognitive dysfunctions. To solve this crisis, medical researchers from around the world have engaged in a desperate search for new treatments to help prevent or treat Alzheimer's disease and other degenerative brain conditions.

For years, American doctors dismissed the value of herbs, preferring instead to prescribe expensive drugs. European doctors, on the other hand, have always prescribed "phytomedicines," or herbal medicines, alongside the pharmaceuticals. And there has been enough research done on these herbs in Europe that physicians in the United States are beginning to take notice.

One of the most impressive bodies of research growing out of this medical challenge to find new treatments consists of several thousand published studies on ginkgo biloba. In China, extracts of the fruit and leaves of the ginkgo tree have been used for more than 5,000 years to treat asthma, cardiovascular diseases, and poor memory. And over the last fifty years, clinical studies have documented the many attributes of this ancient tree herb.

It has been found to alleviate angina pectoris (chest pain) due to coronary artery disease; asthma; depression; intermittent claudication (leg pain due to poor blood flow when walking); macular degeneration; PMS symptoms, including edema (swelling); and tinnitus (ringing in the ears).

It can also:

- Improve memory in both normal adults and those with Alzheimer's disease; pulmonary function; sexual function and desire in both men and women; and visual acuity.

- Inhibit platelet aggregation and the tendency for blood to clot abnormally.

- Reduce or eliminate vertigo (dizziness and loss of stability).

- Reduce elevated blood pressure.

Ginkgo has been able to perform this myriad of beneficial effects because of its antioxidant properties, its ability to enhance blood flow in your arteries and capillaries, and its amazing ability to inhibit the platelet-activating factor (PAF), and thereby prevent abnormal blood clots from forming.

In the following chapters, we will outline the history of this ancient healing herb for you, and examine the growing list of its remarkable health benefits, which includes the ability to boost mental functions, strengthen the cardiovascular system, and fend off the ravages of aging.

CHAPTER 1

DISCOVERY OF A LIVING FOSSIL

If you were to search for a natural compound that could offer protective benefits against the effects of aging, ginkgo would crop up as a most likely candidate. Not only is ginkgo one of the most ancient surviving species in the world—its fossils from the Triassic period date back almost 200 million years—but it is also one of the most long-lived of all plants. There are ginkgo trees that have lived for more than 1,000 years—and they are *still* living.

When the unusually shaped impressions left in ancient shale deposits were first discovered, botanists identified the plant as a gymnosperm, a plant family that includes pines, cedars, and firs. Eventually, fifteen different types of the Ginkgo - aceae tree family were identified, but only from fossil records, so it was believed that all these plants were extinct, the victims of massive climatic changes during the last major ice age.

In the early 1700s, all this changed when Western researchers were stunned to learn that a species of ginkgo had been found *thriving* in China and Asia. The discovery created quite a sensation at the time, particularly as reports about the medicinal uses of this "sacred plant" had begun to surface in the West.

The "Way of Long Life"

The name ginkgo was first given to the newly discovered plant in the early 1700s by a German surgeon working in Asia for the Dutch East India Company. He coined the name ginkgo from the phonetic transcription of a Japanese variation on the Chinese word *yinhsing*, which means "silver apricot." In 1771, the famed Swedish botanist Carolus Linnaeus, recognized as the Father of Taxonomy for his system of classifying plants, renamed the plant ginkgo biloba, ("ginkgo with two lobes") based on the unique division of the leaves into two lobes. The ginkgo tree is also sometimes referred to as the kew or maidenhair tree, because the leaves also bear a likeness to the fronds of maidenhair ferns.

The West soon learned that, in addition to being revered as a sacred plant that was commonly planted around Buddhist temples, the leaves and fruit of the ginkgo tree had been used in traditional Chinese medicine for more than 5,000 years. The discovery of the health-enhancing effects of ginkgo is attributed to the legendary emperor Shen Nong Shi (2,852–2,737 B.C.) who taught primitive farmers to make farming tools and grow crops. Following the "Way of Long Life," Shen Nong devoted himself to the study of various plants and became an expert in the properties of herbal medicines. Since there were no written records at the time, his discoveries were passed down by word of mouth until, almost 2,000 years later during the Han dynasty (206 B.C.–A.D. 220), his teachings were committed to text in the Pen *T'sao Ching* (The Classic of Herbs). Also referred to as the *Materia Medica of Shen Nong*, this earliest recorded text of herbal treatments recommended ginkgo leaves as especially helpful for treating failing memory and relieving the symptoms of asthma and cough.

Shen Nong is also credited with establishing the

concept of opposing principals of nature that are recognized today as the "yin" and "yang" forces of nature. In keeping with this philosophy, ginkgo is considered a dry agent that is best used to counter and balance wet diseases. Then, as now, Chinese healers used the leaves, bark, seeds (or nuts), and the fruits of the ginkgo tree. The leaves were prepared either as a tea or, mixed with rice wine, as a concoction useful for treating angina pectoris, bronchitis, elevated blood fats, fading mental powers, hangovers, or parasites, and for improving blood circulation. The bark was used to treat discharges from the sexual organs, or was applied to the skin as a poultice to prevent infections.

Using the fruit of the ginkgo tree is problematic, as the seeds contain a group of terpene compounds that can irritate the skin and cause a rash. If eaten, the fruit and seeds can irritate the gastrointestinal tract and cause painful spasms and nausea, or can even lead to kidney and liver damage. In order to remove these harmful terpenes, Chinese herbalists learned to prepare ginkgo fruit by boiling it first, then using the seeds to treat conditions such as asthma and diarrhea.

The Ornamental Origins of Ginkgo

The ginkgo was first imported to the United States in 1784 as an attractive ornamental plant that was highly regarded for its extraordinary resistance to insects and disease. Its legendary medical properties were largely unrecognized by the West at the time. The ginkgo is so resistant to damage, in fact, that one ginkgo tree actually survived the atomic bomb dropped on Hiroshima, and is reportedly still alive and growing near the epicenter of the explosion.

One minor problem with the introduction of the ginkgo is that the species is dioecious, meaning that the trees are composed of two distinct sexes that reproduce when windborn pollen from the male tree fertilizes the female tree. Both trees are equally attractive, but the female bears a small fruit with a highly objectionable, foul smell that has been compared to rancid butter or dog droppings. To get around this problem, horticulturists and gardeners simply choose to plant the male ginkgo tree.

Dioecious Trees

"Di" meaning two, is combined with "oecious," from the Greek word oikos for house, to refer to the two houses representing a separate house, or tree, for each of the sexes.

Ginkgo's Unique Chemistry

As ginkgo trees grew in popularity, they spread across urban settings in Europe and America, flourishing in places where other species, less resistant to pollution, diseases, and insects, failed to thrive. Modern research on ginkgo arose from a scientific interest in its adaptive properties, and in the 1950s, German researchers began to study ginkgo in earnest, searching for unknown compounds that might reveal the secret to its unique longevity.

One of the pioneers in ginkgo research was Willmar Schwabe, Ph.D., a West German research - er who set out to isolate the active constituents of the ginkgo leaf and determine if they possessed any medicinal benefits. What Schwabe and his colleagues discovered were a *number of potent compounds that are completely unique to the ginkgo plant and are not found anywhere else in nature.*

Ginkgo's Active Compounds

Flavone Glycosides. Researchers have identified a number of complex molecules in the ginkgo, including a group of special antioxidant compounds known as flavone glycosides, a type of flavonoid (also called bioflavonoids) found in many plants. These compounds act as powerful antioxidants to quench the activity of free radicals—these destructive oxidizing molecules produced normally in the body, and by air pollution, cigarettes, and radiation. Left uncontrolled, free radicals wreak havoc with cells and can damage DNA, setting

Antioxidants
Substances that contribute a spare electron to neutralize damaging free radicals and render them harmless. Antioxidants like vitamins C and E are important for maintaining health and youth.

the stage for degenerative diseases, initiating cancer, and accelerating the aging process. The flavone glycosides isolated from the ginkgo consist of three bioflavonoid compounds known as quercetin, kaempferol, and isorhamnetin. In addition to acting as antioxidants, these flavone glycosides also work together with vitamin C, sparing it from free radical damage and increasing its effectiveness in the body.

One of the most important benefits of the flavonoids is their ability to protect blood vessels. Old age, infection, use of steroid drugs, and nutritional deficiencies common to the elderly all set the stage for weakened blood vessels. These fragile blood vessels are, in turn, more prone to damage, resulting in bruising, even from minor bumps. Flavonoids like those found in Ginkgo have been shown to enhance capillary walls,

Stroke
The third leading cause of death in the U.S. It occurs when a region of the brain loses blood flow, usually from an obstructed blood vessel. Each year about 400,000 cases of stroke and approximately 150,000 deaths from it are reported in the U.S.

thereby protecting vessels from rupture, preventing seepage of blood into surrounding tissues, and reducing inflammation.

Terpene Lactones. A second group of active ingredients isolated from the roots and leaves of ginkgo biloba are several terpene compounds, including terpene lactones. Several studies have found that the terpenes found in the ginkgo protect brain tissues by acting as free radical scavengers outright, while also reducing the formation of free radicals by protecting your brain and nerve cells from the damaging effects of hypoxia (impaired flow of oxygen to the brain). This activity most likely accounts for ginkgo's ability to help in recovering from a stroke.

Cerebral Hypoxia
A condition in which the flow of oxygen to the brain is impaired. The fact that this reduced flow of oxygen does not always involve a diminished flow of blood emphasizes blood's important role in supporting the brain cells outside of delivering oxygen to them.

Terpene lactones also enhance energy by increasing the body's absorption of glucose (blood sugar) and by boosting the body's production of adenosine triphosphate (ATP), the universal energy molecule. This combination of increased glucose intake and ATP production results in increased brain metabolism and physical energy.

Platelet–Activating Factor (PAF) and Ginkgo

Ginkgolide B, one of the terpenes in ginkgo, is particularly important in reducing blood clotting because of its regulatory effects on platelet-activating factor (PAF). Normally, when a wound or injury occurs, the platelets in the blood are stimulated by PAF to become sticky, gather together, and form clots that block the flow of blood. This is a good thing because it protects us from bleeding to death.

But, while a little PAF is necessary for normal

clotting, too much PAF can promote sticky blood, and this can lead to a number of health problems, for example, restricting the flow of blood to the brain, thereby reducing the amount of oxygen it receives. Excess PAF also increases free radical production, damages nerve tissues, initiates rejection of transplanted organs, and promotes inflammation and bronchial constriction. Additionally, the excess platelet aggregation that is triggered by PAF leads to an increased formation of blood clots (thromboses). These can, in turn, lead to heart disease, strokes, and peripheral vascular disease— including intermittent claudication, a painful condition due to impaired circulation in the legs that restricts walking.

Excess production of PAF is believed to be caused by elements of our contemporary lifestyle—a diet high in processed (hydrogenated) fats, chronic exposure to allergens, and stress, for example.

Platelet–Activating Factor
Stimulates platelets in the blood to gather together and form clots to block the flow of blood.

Ginkgolide B has been shown to inhibit PAF and prevent platelet clumping by preventing PAF from binding to the platelets.

The Synergy of Ginkgo

In ancient traditional Chinese medicine, healers used the seeds and leaves of ginkgo to treat their patients. And although the various active compounds isolated from the ginkgo were shown to be effective, researchers determined that these ingredients worked more effectively when taken together, a phenomenon referred to as *synergy*.

Recognizing that the health effects of ginkgo require the right synergistic balance of its active components, German researchers concentrated their efforts on arriving at a standardized extract.

Only by guaranteeing that the final extract contained the correct ratio and potency of the purified active ingredients could a reliable extract be produced for consistent health benefits.

One of the major problems in arriving at a standardized extract is the wide variation and inconsistency in the percentages of active ingredients that may be present in any given crop of harvested ginkgo. Whereas it was traditionally harvested from fallen leaves in ancient China, today's ginkgo is harvested from trees grown on plantations in China, France, and the United States. The leaves are harvested once a year, and only in the fall.

A number of factors can influence the quality and the quantity of the flavonoids and terpene lactones, including the age of the plants, the abundance, or lack, of rainfall, the soil acidity, the growing temperature, and a number of other natural factors. Even under the most strictly controlled growing conditions, the final content of active ingredients can vary enormously.

After years of experimentation, Dr. Willmar Schwabe of Schwabe GmbH, the largest phytomedicine company in Germany, was able to es - tablish a process for producing a guaranteed, standardized extract known as EGb 761. This proc - ess allowed for consistent and reproducible manufacture of a standard potency product that could then be used use in clinical trials. The process starts with the harvesting of green leaves from the male plant in the late summer or early fall, when the flavonoid content is at its highest levels. After harvest, the leaves undergo a complex process involving twenty-seven distinct steps. Over a period of two weeks, fifty pounds of raw leaves are dried and pressed, and the active ingredients are then isolated and balanced.

All this precise work results in a final, purified,

and standardized extract that weighs a mere one pound. Called ginkgo extract, or GBE, it is standardized to contain between 22 and 27 percent ginkgo flavone glycosides, or flavonoids, and 5 and 7 percent terpene lactones. This process has been further standardized. As a result most ginkgo extracts available on the market currently contain ratios of 24 percent ginkgo flavonoids, 6 percent terpene lactones, and 1 percent bilobalide.

CHAPTER 2

GINKGO BILOBA AND THE BRAIN

The human brain is one of the most complex wonders in all of nature. For sheer complexity and processing power, no other organized structure can begin to match this mysterious organ. Composed of some 10 billion neurons and their supportive network, the human brain controls virtually all of our life systems, while generating the flood of thoughts, dreams, and feelings that define our identity and color our very perception of reality. Virtually every thought, concept, opinion, belief, and emotion you have is derived from the millions of chemical and electrical reactions that occur in your brain every minute. And to power all this activity, your brain places a huge demand on your body's energy reserves. Though it accounts for a mere 2 percent of the body's weight, your brain greedily consumes more than 20 percent of your body's available energy in the form of oxygen and glucose. And when your brain activity increases, so too does the demand for energy.

A Matter of Balance

Yet for all of its impressive complexity, your brain is also an extremely delicate organ that depends entirely on the other organs of your body for its existence. The lungs must work continuously to deliver vital oxygen to brain cells, while the liver converts carbohydrates into glucose for energy production.

And your heart and cardiovascular system must work tirelessly to keep blood flowing into your brain to deliver these vital nutrients and remove the resulting waste products. Any condition that interrupts or impairs the flow of blood and oxygen to the brain can cause irreparable damage—and even death—in minutes.

The Aging Brain

Time takes a major toll on the human brain. On average, by age seventy, we lose about 10 percent of our original brain cells from the effects of normal aging. And while our other body tissues, such as the skin and liver have the capacity to regenerate, this trait is not shared by our brain cells—once a brain cell is lost, it is gone forever. With the passage of time, this continual loss of brain cells is further aggravated by damage from by other age-related conditions, such as arteriosclerosis (hardening of the arteries), diabetes, hypertension, and cerebrovascular diseases (CVD), such as cerebrovascular insufficiency, strokes, and multi-infarct dementia (MID).

Brain–Protective Effects of Ginkgo Biloba

Intrigued by historical reports of ginkgo protecting mental functions, European researchers began to study this compound in the 1950s. Initial studies revealed that the unique compounds found only in ginkgo could enhance normal brain functions and aid in the prevention and treatment of a number of brain disorders, including Alzheimer's disease, cerebrovascular insufficiency, and depression, as well as a number of degenerative aging diseases. Their research to date, published in hundreds of studies, has shown that ginkgo biloba is one the safest and most effective agents available for treating age-related mental disorders.

Cerebrovascular Insufficiency

In 1992, a team of German researchers coined a new term—cerebrovascular insufficiency—to describe twelve symptoms common to older people that result from chronically impaired blood flow to the brain. These symptoms include:

- Absent-mindedness
- Anxiety
- Confusion
- Decreased physical performance
- Depression
- Dizziness (vertigo)
- Fatigue
- Lack of energy
- Poor concentration
- Poor memory
- Tinnitus

In addition to causing distress and impairing normal activities, these symptoms are also thought to predict the later onset of dementia (see page 19) or other degenerative diseases.

How Ginkgo Helps Treat Cerebrovascular Insufficiency

Cerebrovascular insufficiency is caused by a reduction in the flow of blood to the brain. This impairment, in turn, reduces the amount of oxygen reaching the cells, which causes an increase in the production of harmful free radicals. This leads to further tissue damage, particularly to the outer membrane of brain neurons.

In Germany, ginkgo has been approved and

licensed for the treatment of cerebral insufficiency based on the positive results of a series of clinical studies. Researchers believe that the positive brain-protecting effects of ginkgo are due to the ability of ginkgo leaf extract to improve blood circulation and oxygen delivery, particularly in the micro-capillaries, and to protect the brain cells against further damage from free radicals. In one study, researchers measured a 57 percent increase in blood flow through capillaries within sixty minutes of giving ginkgo extract to volunteers.

In 1988, in one of the first clinical trials, 166 people over age sixty were given ginkgo as part of a study on the herb's effectiveness in treating cerebral insufficiency. After just three months of treatment, the authors of the study concluded that these test subjects had improved and that the results "confirmed the efficacy of ginkgo extract in cerebral disorders due to aging."

In another early study, reported in 1990, German scientists gave 160 mg of ginkgo extract to a group of sixty hospitalized patients with cerebral insufficiency and depression. Remarkably, the patients given the ginkgo began to show marked improvement after only two weeks, with a significant reduction in many of their symptoms. Over the course of the following four weeks, the researchers noted that eleven of the twelve symptoms listed above had improved significantly in the patients treated with ginkgo extracts, leading to the conclusion that "ginkgo extract can be given to patients with mild to moderate symptoms of cerebral insufficiency."

Placebo Pill
A "sugar pill" or other inert substance used in research studies to exclude the power of suggestion in evaluating the active product or substance being tested.

Again, in 1994, researchers continued to find significant improvements in mental performance after conducting a placebo-controlled, double-blind trial of ninety people with cerebral insufficiency. As in the earlier studies, after only six weeks of treatment with a standardized ginkgo extract, those tested showed marked improvements in their conditions, including significant increases in both short-term memory and concentration.

Dementia, Alzheimer's Disease, and Age-Associated Memory Impairment (AAMI)

Dementia is defined as the loss of intellectual functions. Unlike occasional forgetfulness, dementia is marked by a profound impairment of memory, as well as the loss of additional, complex abilities required for problem-solving, decision-making, spatial orientation, and even the ability to put simple words together to communicate. Dementia is a permanent, progressive disease that mostly affects older people, who may eventually lose the ability to function normally and require round-the-clock care. It is estimated that up to 8 percent of all people over age sixty-five have some form of dementia. That number doubles every five years, leading to an estimate of anywhere from 20 to 50 percent of people in their eighties with dementia. There are close to fifty different causes of dementia, including neurological disorders (Alzheimer's disease), vascular disorders (multi-infarct disease), inherited disorders (Huntington's disease), and infections (viruses such as HIV).

A common factor in all these disorders is a reduced flow of blood and oxygen to the brain. Aside from starving the brain cells of needed fuel, reduced blood flow also increases the production of free radicals, which further damage cell membranes and accelerate brain-cell death. As the number of lost brain cells grows, either from the ravages of age or the debilitating effects of degenerative diseases, mental deterioration continues. Memories begin to fade and the ability to form new thoughts and solve problems is further reduced. Depression, disorientation, incontinence, muscle weakness, speech disturbances, tinnitus (ringing in the ears), tremor, and loss of both visual acuity and coordination also increase as the conditions progress.

Alzheimer's Disease

Alzheimer's disease (also called "senile dementia of the Alzheimer type") is a chronic and progressive, degenerative neurological condition. More than 4 million people in the United States are currently diagnosed with the disease, and it accounts for up to 60 percent of all cases of dementia. Alzheimer's usually appears after age fifty, and from age sixty-five on, the risk of developing the disease doubles every five years. As if these numbers weren't bad enough, they are expected to almost double in the coming decades, placing a further drain on healthcare resources, and leaving almost no family untouched.

While there is currently no cure for Alzheimer's disease, exciting new research shows that ginkgo extract can help in halting the destructive progression of dementia and can offer improvement in the cognitive functions of those with Alzheimer's disease or other forms of dementia.

Alzheimer's disease is associated with a natur-ally occurring key protein called amyloid. In Alz-heimer's, this protein accumulates to form unusual plaques and tangles throughout the brain, leading to dementia, behavioral symptoms, and loss of brain tissues. There is new evidence that the increased production of free radicals seen with aging may be partly responsible for both plaque build-up and the death of brain cells seen in Alzheimer's disease.

Ginkgo Benefits Alzheimer's Patients

Researchers have found that ginkgo can be especially helpful when given to patients at the first sign of symptoms. In one published study, German scientists gave a daily dose of 120 mg of ginkgo to twenty older men and women exhibiting various early symptoms of dementia. The results were dramatic—those receiving ginkgo showed impressive improvements in a variety of clinical tests, as compared to others receiving only a placebo, or dummy pill.

In one large 1996 study, German researchers tested ginkgo extract on a group of 222 people, fifty-five or older, who were diagnosed with a mild to moderate dementia caused either by Alzheimer disease or multi-infarct dementia. They were given either 240 mg of ginkgo biloba extract, twice a day before meals, or a placebo, for the duration of the six-month trial. At the conclusion of the study, the researchers reported those receiving the ginkgo showed a remarkable overall improvement in their condition, including a 300 percent increase in memory and attention, as compared to the others receiving the placebo pills. The researchers concluded their report by stating that, in cases of dementia, ginkgo extract could improve the qual - ity of life while preserving independence and postponing the need for, and expense of, full-time care.

A second German study confirmed the effectiveness of ginkgo in treating people with Alz - heimer's disease. Researchers again divided 216 people, all of them suffering from mild to moderate symptoms of Alzheimer's, into two groups. The first group received 240 mg of ginkgo each day, and the other group received a placebo pill. While this trial lasted for only a month, at its conclusion those receiving the ginkgo again exhibited impressive improvements on tests designed to measure mental functions, showing improvements in alertness and overall mood.

Multi-Infarct Dementia

The second most common cause of dementia in older people is multi-infarct dementia (MID), a condition that accounts for about 15 percent of all cases of dementia. Multi-infarct dementia usually affects people between the ages of sixty and seventy-five, and men are more likely to have multi-infarct dementia than are women. MID is typically caused by a series of mini-strokes, also referred to as transient ischemic attacks (TIAs), that can occur when an artery in the brain either becomes blocked or ruptures. Strokes are generally caused by high blood pressure, high blood cholesterol, diabetes, or heart disease. Of these causes, the most important risk factor for multi-infarct dementia is untreated high blood pressure. In fact, it is extremely rare for a person to develop multi-infarct dementia without also having high blood pressure.

While these mini-strokes may or may not be noticed at the time, the effect on the brain is the same—brain cells become damaged by a lack of oxygen and die. Over time, mini-strokes can begin to destroy the substantial portions of the brain that control speech and visual processing.

As with Alzheimer's disease, ginkgo has been shown to help people with MID by enhancing memory, alertness, and overall quality of life. Additionally, given the underlying disorders that cause blood vessels to rupture, ginkgo can also benefit people with MID by restoring elasticity and strength to their stiff, weakened blood vessels.

CHAPTER 3

GINKGO AND
THE HEART

The human heart is an organ of remarkable precision and reliability. Every minute, this small pear-shaped organ beats seventy-two times to completely recycle approximately five quarts of blood throughout the body. In an average lifetime, the heart will steadily pound out more than 2.5 billion beats, a number most of us remain blissfully ignorant of, until something interrupts this tireless muscle and its life-giving rhythm.

Just as ginkgo supports cerebral blood circulation and increases the flow of oxygen to the brain, it also protects the circulatory system and enhances the delivery of oxygen to the heart and skeletal tissues. Not only does ginkgo improve the overall performance of the circulatory system, but it has also been effective in strengthening weakened blood vessels while restoring some of the elasticity that veins commonly lose with age. In fact, German researchers have shown that taking ginkgo over the long term can protect your heart tissues and reduce your risk of developing heart disease and high blood pressure.

The Circulatory System

The circulatory system carries blood throughout your body. Driven by the pumping actions of the heart, the arteries are the large blood vessels responsible for distributing oxygen and nutrients throughout your body. As the arteries branch off into smaller vessels that continue through the body, the vessels grow smaller and smaller until they reaching the micro-capillaries, which are so small that blood cells must pass through passageways finer than a human hair. As the blood cells deposit their cargo of vital nutrients and oxygen, they exchange them for the cellular waste products they pick up for disposal. Then, as the blood makes its way back up the system, it moves through increasingly larger veins until it reaches the lungs where the waste carbon dioxide is exchanged for fresh oxygen, and the cycle starts all over.

In 1965, the German physician Dr. Willmar Schwabe III identified the beneficial effects of ginkgo on the circulatory system as part of his interest in developing a concentrated extract to be used in clinical study. Schwabe and other researchers found that ginkgo had a number of effects on the human circulatory system. Shortly after ingesting ginkgo, it can be detected in the plasma that accounts for most of the blood's volume. As ginkgo levels rise in the plasma, ginkgo begins to do its work of supporting the myriad cells and tissues that make up the circulatory system.

Ginkgo has improved the circulatory system by helping to strengthen the blood vessels and restore the elasticity that is lost with advancing age. It also acts as a powerful antioxidant that protects the heart and blood vessels from a number of highly reactive and damaging free radicals.

As discussed elsewhere, ginkgo also inhibits the actions of platelet-activating factor (PAF), improving circulation and keeping the blood flowing freely. This enhances the delivery of oxygen to the brain and central nervous system while reducing the risks of both clot (thrombosis) formation and coronary artery spasms that can lead to heart attacks.

Ginkgo and High Blood Pressure

High blood pressure (hypertension) is one of the most common forms of cardiovascular disease, affecting an estimated 25 percent of Americans. Hypertension is associated with atherosclerosis, congestive heart failure, hypertensive renal failure, "myocardial infarction," or heart attack, and stroke. Although hypertension has been extensively studied, more than 90 percent of all cases are referred to as essential hypertension, meaning the cause of the elevated blood pressure is unknown.

A group of Japanese researchers tested the effects of using ginkgo extract to treat hypertension in rats. After feeding ginkgo to the animals for twenty days, the team reported that the rats' high blood pressure was significantly reduced. Additionally, they noted that the rats didn't show any increase in the size of their hearts, a known sign of sustained high blood pressure. Ginkgo's effect appeared to normalize only high blood pressure; there were no changes in the rats with normal blood-pressure levels.

Ginkgo and Arrhythmia

Any change in the regular beating rhythm of the heart is defined as arrhythmia, called tachycardia when the heart beats very fast, and bradycardia when it beats very slowly. Arrhythmias are the result of interference with the electrical pathways that produce the heart's rhythmic muscular contractions. They are responsible for more than 400,000 deaths each year, and are the cause of death for more than two-thirds of heart-disease victims, killing more men in the Western world than any other disease.

While heart disease is a primary cause of arrhythmias, they can also occur in people with no underlying heart disease, caused by such external factors as alcohol, caffeine, cold medications, diet pills, stress, and tobacco.

A large body of research shows that ginkgo leaf extract can protect heart tissues from arrhythmias and the free radical damage caused by the interruption of oxygen and blood flow during a heart attack. In 1994, experimental heart attacks were induced in rat hearts and ginkgo extract not only protected the heart tissues from damage caused by the prolonged lack of oxygen over the forty-minute test period, but it also prevented the occurrence of any arrhythmias normally present following a heart attack.

Heart Attack

Sudden cardiac death is the leading cause of death in the United States, claiming the lives of about 280,000 people each year. It occurs most often in people who have had past heart attacks (myocardial infarctions), but it can also occur in young, healthy individuals. When the heart muscle doesn't get enough oxygen and blood to contract properly and keep pumping blood to the rest of the body, ischemia (lack of oxygen to the heart) results. Ischemia causes problems such as angina pectoris (chest pain), and can lead to cardiac arrest, a fatal heart attack.

Sudden cardiac death also occurs in individuals with no evidence of heart disease. In these people, a silent ischemia caused by coronary artery spasms may be the cause of cardiac arrest. According to investigators, even in the absence of early chest pain and coronary artery disease, transient ischemia can be severe enough to cause life-threatening arrhythmias.

Ginkgo Protects Heart Tissues

Chinese researchers conducted a study to determine if ginkgo could protect heart tissues from the damaging effects of free radicals caused by the lack of oxygen that occurs during heart attacks. In their 1995 study, ginkgo extract was injected directly into the stressed coronary arteries of rabbits suffering from induced oxygen deprivation. Not only did ginkgo protect the heart, but it also significantly reduced the amount of damage to the tissues. According to the study, published in *Biochemistry and Biology International,* these results indicate that the antioxidant properties of ginkgo protected heart tissues from free radicals while helping the damaged tissues to heal from the effects of oxygen deprivation.

A similar study conducted by researchers at the University of California–Berkeley found similar results, indicating that ginkgo is effective in protecting tissues in the heart wall following an interruption in the delivery of oxygen.

Ginkgo Inhibits PAF

One of the greatest health benefits of ginkgo is its ability to increase blood flow—and oxygen delivery—throughout the entire body. One of the primary ingredients in ginkgo is the terpene ginkgolide B and it is able to block the effects of platelet-activating factor (PAF). Under normal circumstances, PAF assists the body in times of trouble by causing platelets to become sticky and come together to form clots that can stem the loss of blood in times of trauma. Unfortunately, when levels of PAF are elevated, due to stress, the consumption of hydrogenated fats, or an exposure to allergens, this life-saving compound can turn into a serious, life-threatening problem. Excess PAF causes blood to thicken too much, increasing the workload for the heart, and restricting the flow of blood throughout the entire body. As if this weren't bad enough, PAF also increases the production of free radicals, causing more damage to the heart and blood vessels. Adding insult to injury, PAF also promotes inflammation which can stress the cardiovascular system and further restrict the delivery of blood and oxygen.

As discussed in Chapter 2, the excess platelet aggregation triggered by PAF also leads to an increase in the formation of blood clots (thromboses) that are involved in heart disease, strokes, and peripheral vascular diseases, such as intermittent claudication (see page 30).

Ginkgo Enhances the Delivery of Blood and Oxygen

The good news is that ginkgo has been effective in inhibiting PAF from binding to platelets and turning blood into a viscous, thick, sludge-like fluid that flows with extreme difficulty. By preventing PAF from binding to platelets, ginkgo also reduces the risks of thrombosis formation and prevents coronary artery spasms, heart attacks, and stroke.

Researchers measured the positive effects of ginkgo on blood viscosity by measuring changes in the speed of blood flowing through the capillaries of ten healthy volunteers. Microcirculation and blood flow were carefully measured before and during a four-hour period following treatment with ginkgo extract. The blood velocity was determined by monitoring circulation in the tiny capillaries located in the nail-fold on the fingernails. One hour after receiving a single dose of 112 mg of ginkgo extract, the researchers found that blood flow had increased by an amazing 57 percent in the test subjects. The researchers found no changes in the quantity of plasma or blood cells. Nor did they find any alterations in blood pressure, capillary diameter, or heart rate. No side effects were reported by any of the patients, and the enhanced blood-circulating effects disappeared after three hours. These findings support many other studies, which show that, by reducing the stickiness of blood cells, which allows an increase in blood flow and the delivery of oxygen to the tissues, ginkgo benefits a variety of conditions.

Another way that ginkgo can help to increase circulation is by its ability to relax (dilate) constricted arteries. A number of animal and human studies have shown that ginkgo is more effective than many standard drugs in relaxing arteries and improving blood circulation. In one human trial, researchers compared ginkgo with standard drugs used to treat vasoconstriction. Twenty-five people were treated with ginkgo and were compared with 300 other people receiving standard medications. By measuring the increase in arteriolar dilation in the big toe of volunteers, the researchers determined that the standard drugs resulted in a 39 percent increase in artery dilation, compared with a 44 percent increase in the group receiving ginkgo.

Ginkgo for Peripheral Arterial Occlusive Disease (PAOD)

Peripheral arterial occlusive disease (PAOD), also known as atherosclerosis obliterans, is a disease caused by thick deposits of plaque forming on the interior lining of the peripheral arteries (atherosclerosis) and the abdominal aorta. In PAOD, the interior diameter of the arteries is so narrowed (generally by 60 percent or more) and constricted that it causes a bottleneck as blood tries to flow out to the arms and legs.

The first symptoms of PAOD often appear as painful aches, tired muscles, and a cramping of the muscles in the arms and legs triggered by exercise. This cramping and pain is referred to as intermittent claudication. As PAOD progresses, walking becomes more difficult due to pain. In time, the pain can grow worse when the limb is elevated, becoming severe enough to prevent sleep. The best treatment for PAOD is usually exercise, but with the extreme pain cause by the condition, this option is not always possible.

Ginkgo for Intermittent Claudication

Given ginkgo's ability to increase blood flow, it's not surprising to learn that painful leg cramping caused by intermittent claudication can be relieved by ginkgo extract. In fact, based on the large number of studies showing ginkgo to be highly effective in treating PAOD and intermittent claudication, both Germany and the World Health Organization have approved ginkgo use as a recognized treatment for these and other related conditions.

Clinical studies have found ginkgo to be highly effective for relieving pain in approximately 75 percent of cases of intermittent claudication. Researchers gauged the effectiveness of ginkgo to increase the flow of blood and oxygen to leg muscles by measuring the maximum distance patients could walk on a standardized treadmill before being forced to stop due to pain. Most studies found that doses between 120 and 240 mg of ginkgo extract led to beneficial effects within about eight weeks, though a more recent study suggests that the higher daily dose of 240 mg of ginkgo is significantly more effective than the lower dose.

Intermittent Claudication

Claudication refers to Emperor Tiberius Claudius Drusus Nero Germanicus who, despite suffering serious birth defects that left him with a lifelong limp, ruled Rome from 41 to 54 AD.

Based on these and numerous other studies on

leg cramps caused by intermittent claudication, researchers believe that, in addition to improving circulation to the peripheral arteries and restoring oxygen, ginkgo also scavenges the free radicals produced by the previously oxygen-deprived muscles.

CHAPTER 4

GINKGO AND SEXUAL ENJOYMENT

In previous chapters we've seen that ginkgo effectively improves blood flow and oxygenation of tissues, protects blood vessels from the ravages of free radicals, and restores elasticity and tone to the entire circulatory system. These same properties are of great importance to the sexual functioning and health of both men and women. In this chapter, we'll discuss the reproductive organs and the role ginkgo plays in enhancing sexual function and enjoyment.

The Poor State of Sexual Satisfaction

The October 1995 *Journal of the American Geriatrics Society* reported that sexual satisfaction and performance in men declines with age. The study by researchers at the Mayo Clinic was based on information obtained from 2,115 men, ranging in age from forty to seventy-nine years. The study evaluated five main factors of sexual health:

- Ability to have erections.

- Changes in sex drive.

- Changes in sexual performance during the previous year.

- Satisfaction with sexual activity.

- Worries or concerns about sexual performance.

The Mayo researchers found that 25 percent of men in their forties were already concerned with their sexual performance. This number rose with age, with 47 percent of men in their seventies reporting they were concerned about their declining sexual function. Key findings of the Mayo study include:

Responses to Questionnaire	Men aged 40–49	Men aged 70–79
Concerned about sexual function	25%	47%
Performance worse than the previous year	10%	30%
Dissatisfied with sexual performance	2%	11%
No sex drive	1%	26%
Difficulty or inability to maintain erections	<1%	27%

The Mayo researchers concluded that decreased satisfaction with sex could be accounted for by age-related increases in erectile dysfunction, decreased libido, and the interaction between erectile dysfunction and decreased libido.

Healthy Sexual Functioning

A normal sexual response in men and women begins in the presence of sexually oriented stimulation. When the mood is right, the body responds by releasing a cascade of chemicals that direct the flow of blood into the sexual organs. In women, this leads to engorgement and lubrication of the organs as the body prepares for intercourse. In men, this rush of blood is directed into a pair of pockets, known as the corpus cavernosum, that run inside the shaft of the penis. This inflow of blood is critical to the enlargement and stiffening of the penis.

This engorgement is triggered by a unique neurotransmitter called nitric oxide (NO). Nitric oxide, in turn, stimulates the production of another signaling enzyme called cyclic guanosine monophosphate, or cGMP for short. Under normal circumstances, cGMP signals the smooth muscles surrounding the arteries of the penis to relax and allow blood to flow into the penis. Any condition that interferes with the signaling of these messenger enzymes can quickly lead to the breakdown of the entire process and cause impotence.

Neurotransmitters
The chemical messengers of the brain. Serotonin, norepinephrine, and dopamine are the best known. Deficiencies in these produce depression. Another one, GABA, is a calming neurotransmitter, and deficiency causes anxiety.

Impotence/Erectile Dysfunction (ED)

According the National Institutes of Health, impotence, or erectile dysfunction, is defined as the inability to attain or sustain an erection adequate for satisfactory sexual intercourse. Experts believe impotence affects between 10 and 15 million American men. In 1985, the National Ambulatory Medical Care Survey counted 525,000 doctor-office visits for erectile dysfunction, and that number has greatly increased since then.

Impotence usually has a physical cause, such as disease, injury, or drug side effects. Any disorder that impairs blood flow in the penis has the potential to cause impotence. It occurs as men age: about 5 percent of men at age forty, and between 15 and 25 percent of men at age sixty-five expe-rience impotence. Yet, it is not an inevitable part of aging.

Viagra

In 1998, the FDA approved the prescription drug Viagra (sildenafil citrate) as a treatment for men suffering from nonorganic impotence due to conditions such as diabetes, radical prostatectomy, spinal cord injury, and vascular disease.

Viagra was originally investigated as a potential anti-angina medication based on its ability to release nitric oxide and increase blood flow to the heart. Although Viagra failed as a heart medication, researchers in London noted that many of the men in the clinical trials reported the frequent occurrence of unaccustomed erections and improved sexual performance. Following this serendipitous finding (and five years of clinical trials), Viagra was finally granted approval as a treatment for men who had difficulty achieving erections because of conditions such as diabetes, radical prostatectomy, spinal cord injury, and vascular disease.

Enzymes
Enzymes are protein structures that act as catalysts to promote the billions of biochemical reactions necessary for virtually all life processes.

Viagra was found to help men achieve and maintain erections by (1) enhancing the effects of the neurotransmitter nitric oxide (NO), and (2) maintaining higher levels of the enzyme cGMP, the two key players in penile erection. Viagra does this by selectively inhibiting the enzymes that destroy cGMP, leading to ele-vated cGMP levels. This, in turn, increases blood flow to the genitals and leads to stronger erections and intensified sensation.

Viagra was found to help 80 percent of men suffering from nonorganic impotence. Additionally, Viagra also seems to enhance sexual performance and enjoyment, and reduce the latent period between erections, even in men who have no dysfunction.

Women and Viagra

Viagra has also gained a reputation with women, which makes sense when one considers that the clitoris, which is structurally similar to the penis, becomes engorged with blood during sexual arousal. Viagra may provide similar benefits to women, by stimulating the release of NO to encourage the flow of blood and enhance their sexual sensation and orgasmic enjoyment.

Serious Side Effects of Viagra

While Viagra is effective for millions of men, the side effects for many—facial flushing, headaches, and indigestion—are too troublesome for continued enjoyment. And, more seriously, soon after its introduction, vision problems began to surface in men taking viagra, leading to warnings for people with retinal eye conditions, such as macular degeneration or retinitis pigmentosa, to use the drug with caution.

In addition to eye problems, both the FDA and the manufacturer began to issue warnings against taking Viagra with any nitrate-based cardiac medications (that is, sublingual nitroglycerin tablets, nitroglycerin patches, and the like). Doctors were warned that heart patients should not be treated with nitroglycerin if the patient had used Viagra in the previous twenty-four hours. Additionally, the manufacturer reported several cases where patients who received both drugs died after developing irreversible hypotension (a severe drop in blood pressure).

As safety issues with Viagra began to arise, researchers once again began to seek out safer alternatives for treating impotence.

Ginkgo Offers a Safer Alternative

Many current pharmaceuticals have evolved from

the historical search for herbal compounds to cure or reverse sexual dysfunction. Often, traditional nostrums rely on purely magical (placebo) effects, such as the phallic-influenced belief in the effect of rhinoceros horn—which, in fact, offers no benefit to humans and is fatal for the unfortunate rhino. Conversely, many plant-based traditional treatments, using herbs such as damiana, maca, muira puama, tribulus, and yohimbe, have been explored for their effectiveness in treating sexual dysfunction.

Armed with the fresh body of knowledge revealed by the success of Viagra, researchers once again turned their attentions to the ginkgo extract.

Ginkgo Enhances Sexual Function

Recognizing that circulatory problems are a major cause of impotence, it comes as no surprise that ginkgo has been effective in treating erectile dysfunction caused by impaired blood flow. In one study, ginkgo was found effective in improving erectile dysfunction in a group of impotent males taking 60 mg of ginkgo extract for six months. Researchers suggested that ginkgo worked by stimulating the release of nitric oxide (NO), which, as described above, signals the blood vessels to dilate and sends blood to the corpus cavernosum to achieve and maintain an erection.

Ginkgo's positive effects on impotence were further established by a second study, reported in the *Journal of Urology*, in which researchers found that ginkgo was highly effective in helping men achieve and maintain erections. What was remarkable about this study is that it was involved sixty men who had previously failed to respond to papaverine, an injectable prescription medication commonly used to treat male sexual dysfunction. The men were given ginkgo extract, 60 mg per day, for up to eighteen months. The first signs of improvement were noticed after only six weeks. After six months of therapy, 50 percent of the men were able to achieve erections and engage in sex. By the end of the study, fully 95 percent of the men receiving ginkgo extract showed significant improvements in penile blood flow. According to the study authors, the improvements were due to the direct effect of ginkgo extract to enhance blood flow in arteries and veins.

Ginkgo and Antidepressant–Induced Sexual Problems

Millions of people have been helped by a variety of medications commonly used to treat clinical depression. Unfortunately many antidepressants, especially the class of drugs known as selective serotonin reuptake inhibitors (SSRIs), have a negative effects on a person's sexual libido and satisfaction. Antidepressant-related sexual problems include decreased sexual drive, delayed ejaculation, and difficulty achieving orgasm. It's been estimated that sexual problems related to antidepressants occur in more than 70 percent of patients, though embarrassment leads to under - reporting by both doctors and patients.

Ginkgo has been an effective treatment for sexual problems related to the use of the commonly prescribed antidepressant drugs. Researchers tested the effects of ginkgo extract on a group of thirty men and thirty-three women who were suffering from sexual side effects attributed to the use of antidepressant drugs, such as the selective serotonin reuptake inhibitors (SSRIs). Sexual side effects ranged from decreased libido and erectile difficulties to delayed or inhibited orgasm.

Each person received ginkgo extract in doses ranging from 80–120 mg daily. After only four weeks, 84 percent of those tested reported positive results in all phases of the sexual response cycle. A major point of interest with this study is that women responded better than men, with 91 percent of the women reporting improvements in the sexual response, as compared to 76 percent of the men indicating success. No adverse effects were reported and the use of ginkgo biloba appeared to be compatible with antidepressant therapy. As in most other studies, the researchers reported that many subjects also experienced improved cognitive functioning, mental clarity, and memory, and increased energy. And, as with other studies on ginkgo and sexual dysfunction, the researchers of the study attributed the success to ginkgo's ability to aid circulatory function.

Ginkgo as an Aphrodisiac?

Given ginkgo's proven ability to dilate blood vessels and improve blood flow to the penis, it is not surprising to note that many aphrodisiac formulas contain ginkgo extract. According to Dr. Stephen Karch, a specialist in cardiac pathology and author of *The Consumer's Guide to Herbal Medicine,* ancient Chinese herbalists referred to ginkgo as an aphrodisiac. Karch reports that ginkgo enhances nitric oxide (NO) production. Nitric oxide is the primary messenger molecule that is affected by Viagra, and is the key factor in helping achieve erections by informing certain blood vessels to relax.

CHAPTER 5

GINKGO AND VISION

Ginkgo has been studied extensively for its ability to treat a wide variety of vision-related conditions. Age-related cataracts, glaucoma, macular degeneration, and diabetic retinopathy are among the leading causes for loss of vision. Unfortunately, standard medical approaches to preserving sight haven't offered much hope for treatment of these blinding eye diseases. Ginkgo is believed to benefit these and other vision problems by preventing the damage caused by free radical activity and by enhancing the delivery of blood and oxygen to the retina to help repair tissues.

The Eye as a Camera

The inside of the eye has been compared to a camera. Light enters through the lens and is focused onto the retina, a layer of tightly packed and highly sensitive photoreceptors that line the interior back surface of the eyeball. The retina contains millions of light-sensitive cells, called rods and cones, that enable us to pick out colors and fine details. When light hits any of these cells, there is a biochemical reaction to the varying intensities of light and color. The cells then transmit electrical signals along nerve cells to the brain where all the information is assembled and processed to form a picture that we experience as vision.

The cells lining the retina expend a great deal

of energy, and require a constant supply of oxygen, glucose, and other nutrients. Consequently, the retina is supplied by a dense tangle of blood vessels that provide one of the highest rates of blood flow found anywhere in the body.

The retina is a delicate structure that is highly vulnerable to oxidative damage from free radicals. The tissues of the retina are also rich in polyunsaturated fatty acids, which are particularly attractive to free radicals.

Ginkgo for Healthy Vision

Because ginkgo extract is such a potent free radical scavenger, scientists believed it would support healthy vision by preventing the age-related accumulation of free radical damage that is commonly blamed for eye diseases, such as macular degeneration and diabetic retinopathy.

To test their theory, German scientists studied ginkgo's protective effects on the retinas of twenty-five older people. They found that just 160 mg per day of the extract resulted in dramatically improved vision for all of these subjects after only four weeks of treatment. According to the researchers, the ginkgo caused a "significant increase in retinal sensitivity."

Ongoing studies show that the greater the damage to retinal tissues, the more profound an effect the ginkgo has on improving vision. A significant finding was that ginkgo had virtually no side effects and that normal retinal functions were unaffected, proving the safety of the herb. These studies showed that ginkgo was not only effective in improving vision, but, in cases where the vision was damaged by poor circulation, the damage could be significantly reversed.

Another form of age-related eye deficiency is the gradual loss of an ability to tell the difference between certain colors. This skill peaks in middle age and, like so many other human abilities, declines with age, reducing once-vibrant colors to more muted shades of pastel or gray.

Again, research has found that ginkgo can help here. After French scientists gave twenty-nine older volunteers ginkgo extract for six months, tests revealed that their ability to distinguish differences in shades of color had improved.

Diabetic Retinopathy

Diabetic retinopathy is a serious complication of diabetes that damages the small blood vessels of the retina. People with diabetes are at increased risk of developing eye problems, such as cataracts and glaucoma, but diabetic retinopathy is the number one vision threat for diabetic patients, affecting half of all diabetics in America. If left untreated, about half of those with the advanced form, proliferative retinopathy, will become blind within five years, compared to just 5 percent of those who receive treatment.

In the early stages of the disease—called non-proliferative, or background retinopathy—the small blood vessels of the retina weaken and develop bulges (micro-aneurysms) that can leak blood (hemorrhage) or fluid (exudates) into the surrounding tissues. The person's vision is rarely affected during this stage of retinopathy.

In the advanced, proliferative stage of retinopathy, circulation problems resulting from damaged and narrowed blood vessels cause the retina to become oxygen-deprived. To cope with this, the circulatory system attempts to maintain adequate oxygen levels within the retina by forming fragile new blood vessels that can grow on the retina and extend into the vitreous (the jellylike substance inside the back of the eye).

These fragile vessels can rupture and release blood into the interior of the eye, leading to blurred vision or temporary blindness. The resulting formation of scar tissue here can eventually pull the retina away from the back of the eye (retinal detachment), and lead to permanent vision loss. In addition, at any stage of retinopathy, a condition called macular edema can occur. This is a severe blurring of the vision when fluid accumulates around the macula, which is the most sensitive part of the retina, and the one that is crucial for seeing fine detail.

Retinal Detachment

A retinal detachment occurs when the retina is pulled away from the back of the eye, leading to blurred vision and blindness if not treated.

All people with diabetes—including type I (juvenile onset) and type II (adult onset)—are at risk for developing diabetic retinopathy. Controlling diabetes is no guarantee that you will not develop retinopathy, either, so you must always be on guard. Pregnant women with diabetes are more prone to developing diabetic retinopathy, so dilated eye examinations each trimester are recommended for these women, to protect their vision.

In standard conventional medicine, both macular edema and peripheral retinopathy are treated with focal laser photocoagulation, a procedure that uses a laser in the vicinity of the macula to seal the leaking blood vessels. Pan-retinal photocoagulation is another, related procedure used by conventional medicine to minimize proliferative retinopathy. It works by targeting hundreds of spots across the retina in order to stop the bleeding from abnormal new vessels and prevent their further growth.

Ginkgo and Retinopathy

A number of experimental studies suggest that

ginkgo extracts are potentially useful for treating retinal damage induced by a variety of disorders. Many of the results point to antioxidants as the reason for the protective effects of the extract. In addition, it is suspected that ginkgo's ability to inhibit the platelet-activating factor (PAF), is involved in protecting eye tissues from retinopathy, since ginkgolide B, a known PAF antagonist, has been shown to reduce experimentally induced retinal lesions in animals.

In 1992, a group of researchers tested ginkgo to see if it could protect retinal tissues from the destructive effects of free radicals involved in diabetic retinopathy. After conducting several experimental studies to establish that free radicals were indeed an important cause of the damage seen in diabetic retinopathy, they tested a group of diabetic rats that were fed ginkgo (100 mg/kg) daily for two months. At the end of the study, they concluded that ginkgo was a highly effective free radical scavenger that prevented the retinopathy associated with diabetes.

Human studies also support the use of ginkgo extract in treating retinopathy. In one double-blind trial, researchers gave daily doses of 160 mg of a standardized ginkgo extract to a small group of people with mild diabetic retinopathy. After six months, these volunteers had a noticeable improvement of their pre-existing impaired vision.

Double-Blind Study

In double-blind studies, neither the researchers nor the study participants are aware of who is taking which product until the end when the code is broken and the results are tallied.

A second double-blind, placebo-controlled trial, using twenty-nine people with early diabetic retinopathy, found similar protective effects. Half of the participants (fourteen) were given 80 mg per day of ginkgo extract for six months, while the other half (fifteen) received a placebo. At the end of the trial, those who had received the ginkgo extract showed a small but significant increase in their color vision, indicating a reversal of retinal damage, while the vision of the group receiving the placebo was worse than at the beginning of the study.

Macular Degeneration

Macular degeneration is a term for a group of disorders that all involve the slow destruction of the macula, the central region of the retina. Most cases of macular degeneration occur in people over age sixty and are therefore referred to as age-related macular degeneration (ARMD). ARMD is a major cause of blindness affecting up to 15 million people over age sixty.

As we said, the macula is a crucial part of the center of the retina. It contains an extraordinary array of photosensitive cells that enable us to perceive color and fine details. In ARMD, the macula slowly deteriorates, eventually leading to almost complete blindness in our central visual field and leaving us with only the very edges of peripheral vision. Mainstream medicine can only offer laser surgery or radiation as last-ditch solutions to halting any further loss of vision after the disease has progressed to the point of imminent blindness.

Macular degeneration causes different symptoms in different people, and in its early stages there may be few noticeable changes in vision. Often there is only loss of vision in one eye while the other eye continues to see well for many years. But when both eyes are affected, reading and close-up work can become difficult.

Ginkgo and ARMD

ARMD, like atherosclerosis, is a disease caused by

poor circulation. If blood flow is affected by atherosclerosis, diabetes, or any other age-related health problem, the macula slowly atrophies and dies. This process is further hastened by the accelerated production of free radicals that accumulate in the retina when there is reduced blood flow.

Atherosclerosis
A disease in which arteries are narrowed by cholesterol-rich plaque. Risk factors include elevated cholesterol and triglyceride levels, high blood pressure, and cigarette smoking.

Smoking contributes to the progression of ARMD by reducing the supply of blood, narrowing the blood vessels, and thickening the blood. A high-fat, high cholesterol diet leading to fatty plaque deposits in the macular vessels also hampers blood flow. Additionally, a shortage of antioxidants may also increase the tendency for ARMD.

Armed with these insights, scientists speculated that ginkgo extract might slow the progression of ARMD by increasing blood flow to the retina and by halting the free radical damage to the photosensitive cells. To test this theory, researchers conducted a double-blind trial in 1988 to see if the antioxidant and circulatory effects of ginkgo extract could reverse or halt the progression of macular degeneration. Twenty volunteers were given either 160 mg of ginkgo extract, or a placebo pill, every day for six months. At the end of the study, the group receiving ginkgo showed significant improvements in their long-distance visual focus. There was no improvement in the group receiving the dummy pill.

Glaucoma: The "Sneak Thief of Sight"

According to the American Academy of Ophthalmology (AAO), more than 1 million people in the

United States are at risk for going blind because they don't know they have glaucoma. Once thought of as a single disease, glaucoma is actually the term for damage to the optic nerves (the bundle of nerve fibers that carries information from the eye to the brain) caused by elevated pressure inside the eye. It is estimated that about 50 million people worldwide have impaired vision, if not complete blindness, from glaucoma. In the United States, about 300,000 new cases are diagnosed each year, adding to the more than 3 million cases already on record.

Glaucoma is called the "sneak thief of sight" because it strikes without obvious symptoms. People with glaucoma are usually unaware of it until they have a serious loss of vision. In fact, about half of those who have glaucoma do not know it. Currently, that damage cannot be reversed.

While there are usually no warning signs, some symptoms may occur in the later stages of the disease, such as a loss of peripheral vision, difficulty focusing on close work, seeing halos around lights, and frequent changes of prescription glasses. Unfortunately, though, once the vision is lost, it is gone forever.

African Americans are at a higher risk of developing glaucoma than other racial groups. Others at risk include:

- Anyone with a close relative who has glaucoma.

- Seniors.

- Those with diabetes.

- Those who have been taking steroid medication for a long time.

Ginkgo to the Rescue for Glaucoma

Ginkgo extract can increase the circulation of

blood to the eyes, and in some cases, it can help lower the intraocular pressure in the eyes. In one double-blind, placebo-controlled study of older people with macular degeneration, there was a significant improvement in their vision following treatment with ginkgo extract.

In 1999, there was a second study to test the therapeutic effects of ginkgo extract on people with glaucoma. Eleven healthy volunteers were treated with either 40 mg of ginkgo extract, or a placebo, three times daily for two days. Using Doppler imaging, a technique that uses a low-power laser beam, to measure the flow of blood in the eyes before and after treatment, the researchers found a significant increase in blood flow in the main eye artery in those receiving ginkgo. No change was noted in the placebo group. The results indicate that ginkgo effectively increased the blood flow in the eyes which helped lower the intraocular pressure, thereby slowing the progression of the disease.

Ginkgo Protects against UV–Induced Eye Damage

You have only one pair of eyes, and protecting them from excess sunlight is every bit as important as protecting your skin. Overexposure to intense ultraviolet (UV) radiation produced by the sun can cause damage to the cornea, leading to a painful condition known as photokeratitis. Ultraviolet radiation also contributes to the development of other serious eye disorders, including cataracts, degenerative corneal changes, and skin cancer around the eye. It may also contribute to age-related macular degeneration.

Results from a dozen studies over the last ten years suggest that spending time in direct sunlight without wearing proper eye protection can significantly increase your chances of developing any of these serious eye diseases.

UV actually refers to three types of ultraviolet light—UV-A, UV-B, and UV-C. The milder form of radiation, UV-C rays, are normally screened out by the ozone layer and don't present much of an immediate health threat. The more powerful UV-A rays are composed of longer wavelength radiation that causes skin tanning and premature skin aging. UV-A rays can reach the retina, and long-term exposure to them may greatly increase your incidence of macular degeneration. UV-B light, the active, shorter wavelengths of radiation, are responsible for blistering sunburns and skin cancer, and they cause the greatest damage to your eyes.

Ginkgo can protect your retina from damaging exposure to sunlight. Researchers found that when experimental rats were fed ginkgo two to four weeks prior to exposure to intense light, the antioxidant activity of the ginkgo protected the retinal cells from oxidative damage. The untreated animals fared poorly. There was extensive damage to their retinal tissues, leading to a loss of photoreceptors, fragmentation of their cells, and extensive cell death in their maculas. Ginkgo also prevented a reduction in the thickness of the retinal layer, suggesting that ginkgo was effective in protecting the cells from free radical damage, both from sunlight and as a response by the body's immune system.

> **Immune System**
>
> The immune system is composed of a complex combination of responses that fight invaders, such as bacteria and viruses.

Ginkgo and Cataracts

Cataracts, a cloudiness of the lens inside the eyes that occurs over a period of many years, are a major cause of visual impairment and blindness worldwide. Studies have implicated UV radiation in the development of cataracts, and have also shown that certain types of cataracts are linked to a history of higher exposure to UV rays, especially UV-B radiation.

Since UV-B radiation is reflected off bright surfaces, such as sand, snow, and water, the risk is particularly high on the beach, in mountain areas, or while boating. The risk is greatest during the midday hours, during the summer months, and at high altitudes any time of year. Ultraviolet radiation levels also increase as you get nearer the equator, so residents in the equatorial countries and parts of Northern Australia are at greater risk than those living in temperate zones.

Since the human lens absorbs UV radiation, individuals who have cataract surgery are at increased risk of retinal damage from sunlight. And people with retinal dystrophies or other chronic retinal conditions may be at an even greater risk since their retinas may be less resilient to normal exposure levels to begin with.

Ginkgo is believed to be protective because it helps prevent the free radical damage caused by lifelong exposure to sunlight. To date, there has been only one small study conducted with ginkgo and cataracts, but it showed promising benefits. More research is being done in this area.

CHAPTER 6

GINKGO AND HEARING DISORDERS

More than 28 million Americans are deaf or have hearing problems, and 30 million more are at risk of losing their hearing from exposure to dangerous levels of noise. Our ears can detect frequencies ranging from 20 Hz to 20,000 Hz, but it is most sensitive to the sounds commonly used for speech, which range from 1500 Hz to 3000 Hz. Hearing deficits can occur for the following reasons:

• Sound waves are not properly conducted to the cochlea in the ear.

• Scar tissue hampers the cochlear nerves.

• Sound processing in the brain is damaged.

Cochlea

The cochlea, so named for its snaillike spiral shape, transmits auditory information to the part of the brain that processes sound.

Hearing losses can range from a minor nuisance, such as a difficulty understanding light conversation, or enjoying a full range of musical notes, to total deafness. Older people are the largest group of Americans with hearing loss. It affects 30 to 35 percent of the United States population over age age sixty-five, and up to 50 percent of the population over eighty-five. But hearing problems are not exclusive to these groups—in the United States about 1 million school-age children have some degree of hearing loss or total deafness. The most common cause of hearing loss in children is otitis media (middle ear infection) and that primarily affects infants and young children.

Hearing affects how we communicate and interact with the world around us. With the seemingly inevitable age-related loss of hearing, older people can become withdrawn in an attempt to avoid the embarrassment and frustration of appearing confused, unresponsive, or uncooperative. This isolation often leads to depression as well.

During the last decade, important progress has been made in understanding the human ear and the hearing processes. In this chapter, we will discuss some positive studies that have been conducted on ginkgo and hearing disorders, such as deafness, tinnitus, and vertigo, that are associated with cerebral insufficiency or a reduction in the flow of blood to the inner ear.

Ginkgo Improves Hearing in Sudden Deafness

A number of studies have shown that ginkgo is highly effective in improving hearing, particularly when hearing losses are caused by very loud sounds. Researchers believe that, by restoring circulation to the tiny blood vessels damaged by a lack of oxygen, ginkgo protects and restores function to the cells and blood vessels in the ear.

A French study in 1986 found that ginkgo effectively improved the hearing in the test subjects who all had acute cochlear deafness. This type of deafness, which keeps sound vibrations from getting to the brain, is the result of an insufficient flow of blood to the cochlea. Eighteen people in this double-blind trial received either 320 mg of ginkgo extract daily for thirty days, or nicergoline (Semion®), a migraine medication that acts as a vasodilator. While both groups showed improvements, 52 percent of those receiving the ginkgo showed significant improvements in their hearing, compared to only 35 percent in the nicergoline group.

In a second clinical study in 1986, German researchers evaluated a group of fifty-nine people with sudden deafness who were being treated with ginkgo extract. After nine weeks, 59 percent of these test subjects rated their improvement in hearing from good to very good. Of the thirty-three people who initially reported having ringing in the ears (tinnitus), 36 percent said their symptoms were completely resolved, and 15 percent said they were substantially reduced.

Vasodilator
A vasodilator relaxes the blood-vessel walls, causing them to dilate, and allowing blood, oxygen, and nutrients to pass through them more easily.

Tinnitus

An estimated 50 million Americans suffer from some form of tinnitus (pronounced tǐn′-ǐ-tǐs), a medical term for a ringing in the ears. Most people with tinnitus report this as a constant, nonstop ringing noise, while others describe hearing an assortment of hissing, chirping, or clicking sounds. Tinnitus is not a disease, but is a very persistent disturbance that rarely lets up except for an occasional reduction in the loudness of the noise levels.

Tinnitus is most commomly caused by constant exposure to loud noises. Other conditions that can trigger tinnitus include ear, sinus, and respiratory infections, severe head trauma, some types of tumors, and wax build-up. Certain drugs, such as aspirin, birth control pills, quinine, and some antibiotics, can magnify the effects of tinnitus.

Ginkgo and Tinnitus

Although currently there is no cure or effective medical treatment for tinnitus, hearing aids and white noise audiotapes can offer some relief. But a systematic review of nineteen clinical studies on the subject found that ginkgo extract offered a significant reduction in tinnitus symptoms, particularly if the treatments got started soon after the symptoms were first detected.

In a 1986 double-blind study, French researchers treated 103 people for tinnitus with either 320 mg of ginkgo extract, or a placebo. While only 24.4 percent of those receiving the placebo showed improvement, 40 percent of those receiving the ginkgo reported marked relief from their symptoms. The rest of the ginkgo group also derived varying degrees of benefits from it.

Vertigo and Dizziness

Like tinnitus, vertigo and dizziness are not diseases, but they are very unpleasant symptoms of underlying problems that affect balance. Vertigo is often described as a spinning or rotary motion. Some people say vertigo makes them feel as if they are spinning. Others say they are standing still, but the environment around them is rotating. Still others feel they are being pushed or pulled off balance.

Dizziness is similar to vertigo, but with added symptoms, such as disorientation, fuzzy vision, lightheadedness, nausea, sweating, and fainting.

Disruptions of Motion and Balance

Vertigo and dizziness can be symptoms of an underlying disorder affecting our vestibular system, the one responsible for helping us maintain our senses of motion and balance. It works by monitoring the direction and speed of our head movements and transmitting this information to special-ized organs inside the ear before passing it on to different parts of our brain, mainly the cerebellum, for final processing. In the brain, this information on balance and motion is integrated with the sensory information received from our eyes, ears, legs, and arms to help it figure out our body's position in space.

Cerebellum
The cerebellum is the part of the brain that coordinates move-ment so we can maintain balance, grasp objects accurately, and keep our eyes focused during motion, or while walking.

Ginkgo can help control ver-tigo and dizziness, once again by promoting the flow of blood, this time to aid the brain in accurately receiving and evaluating sen-sory information.

Motion and Balance Disorders and Ginkgo

The effects of ginkgo leaf extract on motion and balance (vestibular) disorders has been examined in animals. When researchers treated cats with ginkgo extract, their vestibular damage was re-versed, and the cats had their balance completely restored. And, as little as four weeks of treatment with ginkgo extract improved the cochlear blood flow in rats and adult guinea pigs, and helped them recover from balance and motion disturbances.

These findings also apply in studies on humans. In one 1985 multi-center trial, seventy people with vertigo were given either 160 mg of ginkgo, or a placebo, daily for three months. In terms of inten-sity, frequency, and duration of the vertigo symp-toms, the group treated with ginkgo extract showed a greater improvement than the placebo group. These improvements were noticed in as lit-tle as one month and they increased over the full three months of the trial. The outcome of this remarkable trial was that, by the end of the study, 47 percent of those treated with the ginkgo extract were completely free of vertigo symptoms, while only 18 percent of those who received the placebos were symptom-free.

Based on the success of these studies, it seems worthwhile to consider taking ginkgo extract at the first sign of any problems you may have with balance or dizziness.

CHAPTER 7

GINKGO'S OTHER
HEALTH BENEFITS

In addition to its well-documented and clinically proven abilities to improve circulation and cognitive performance, researchers around the world continue to be impressed by the growing list of additional health properties being attributed to ginkgo.

In this chapter, we will briefly examine some recent studies on these other conditions that continue to impress researchers.

Ginkgo and Premenstrual Syndrome (PMS)

In 1931, scientists investigating problems of menstruation identified a group of symptoms that typically start a week or so prior to menstruation. They labeled the condition premenstrual tension (PMT), an umbrella term for the depression, extreme fatigue, and irritability that many women experienced during the premenstrual period. As research continued, it became evident that PMT was only part of a syndrome of more than 100 documented symptoms, so the name was changed to premenstrual syndrome (PMS). PMS affects up to 90 percent of all women at some point during their lives, some so severely that they cannot go about their daily tasks.

The most commonly reported symptoms of PMS are bloating, breast swelling or tenderness, cravings for sweets, depression, fatigue, head-aches, irritability, loss of sex drive, and weight gain. Various treatments, including vitamins, minerals, and hormones, such as progesterone, have been shown to help some women cope with many symptoms of PMS.

Ginkgo and Fluid Retention

Fluid retention syndrome, medically referred to as cyclic edema, is a condition seen primarily in young women just before they menstruate. The symptoms include tissue swelling (edema) in the legs and abdomen after sitting or standing for periods of time, or heavy swelling of the face and eyelids when lying down, causing moderate discomfort. Other symptoms include aching, carpal tunnel syndrome, headaches, muscle and joint pains, and stiffness. The condition is thought to be caused by fluids leaking from the blood out into the surrounding tissues. It is often seen in existing premenstrual syndrome and it can worsen PMS symptoms.

Edema

Edema is caused by an accumulation of fluid between the cells that leads to swelling. Edema is most often seen in the lower legs, the feet, and around the eyes.

In a 1993 French study, researchers discovered that ginkgo extract is highly effective in relieving the fluid retention associated with cyclic edema. Ten women with severe cases were treated with 160–200 mg of ginkgo extract daily for two months. Of the ten, three women showed a complete elimination of their swelling and, in fact, never experienced the problem again. The other participants improved significantly, and tests showed that the fluid leakage had been stopped completely.

In a continuation of this study, researchers treated five women who had even greater fluid retention with an intravenous infusion of 200–300 mg of ginkgo extract once a day. After five days, each of the women had lost between four and ten pounds of water weight.

Ginkgo and PMS Symptoms

A larger study confirmed the early findings of ginkgo's effects on fluid retention, showing that ginkgo extract was effective in relieving other symptoms commonly seen in PMS. French researchers conducted the trial with 165 women, eighteen to forty-five years old, who reported experiencing at least three consecutive cycles of discomfort related to PMS. The women were divided into two groups and given daily doses of either ginkgo extract, or a placebo. After two months, the ginkgo was found to be highly effective in treating their other PMS symptoms, particularly in relieving their breast symptoms and improving their moods.

Ginkgo and Depression

Statistics show that depression affects about 17 million Americans, with 25 percent of the population likely to suffer diagnosable depression during their lifetime. Prescription antidepressants are the conventional treatment, with their harmful side effects, and potential for overdose.

German researchers have investigated the effectiveness of ginkgo for treating people who are depressed. They treated forty people, aged fifty-one to seventy-eight, who were diagnosed with mild-to-moderate cerebral dysfunctions that were combined with episodes of depression. All of these people had failed to respond to conventional antidepressant medications. They continued to take their medications while also receiving either 80 mg of ginkgo three times a day or a placebo. In the ginkgo group, there was a 50 percent reduction in the severity of depression after four weeks, and a 68 percent reduction after eight weeks. Overall, these people were significantly more motivated, more optimistic, and happier. By contrast, those receiving the placebo showed a less than 10 percent improvement in their depression symptoms at both four and eight weeks.

As a result of the impressive effects ginkgo has on depression, the German Ministry of Health Committee for Herbal Remedies has approved the use of ginkgo extract for improving mood and mental processes.

Ginkgo and Radiation

Following the 1986 Chernobyl disaster in the Ukraine, researchers detected compounds that damaged chromosomes in the plasma of thirty people assigned to cleaning up and shutting down the Chernobyl nuclear plant after it malfunctioned. This genetic damage meant that the workers were at a greatly increased risk for developing cancer. Medical researchers gave the workers 40 mg of ginkgo, three times a day, in the hope that the same antioxidant effects that had preserved the surviving ginkgo tree at Hiroshima would reduce the dangerous compounds in the serum of the Chernobyl workers.

After eight weeks of treatment, the researchers reported that these dangerous compounds had been reduced significantly, to the same levels as people who had not been exposed to high levels of radiation. These levels were maintained for at least seven months after taking the herb. After seven months, researchers measured a return of the serum markers showing damage, suggesting that treatment with ginkgo needed to be extended, possibly for the life of the patients.

Ginkgo and Sunburn

Based on its powerful antioxidant properties and proven ability to protect the body against the ravages of high radiation exposure, it isn't surprising that ginkgo also protects against sunburn and prevents sun damage. This is because it increases circulation to the skin, which acts to protect and stabilize collagen, which, in turn, protects against the ravages of solar radiation from the sun. Experiments suggest that, once the skin has had sun damage, ginkgo extract can speed its recovery while helping to reduce the pain of sunburn.

Ginkgo and Hepatitis B

Hepatitis B (HBV) is a chronic liver infection that spreads from person to person through blood transfusions and sexual contact. HBV infection can cause severe liver disease, including liver failure (cirrhosis) and liver cancer. HBV affects one out of every twenty people living in the United States, and each year more than 5,000 people die from hepatitis-B-related liver disease.

Chinese researchers tested ginkgo, known to be a powerful anti-inflammatory, to see if it could help control the liver inflammation that occurs with chronic hepatitis infection. The researchers gave ginkgo to eighty-six patients with chronic, persistent and active HBV, with early fibrosis (scarring) confirmed by liver biopsy. After three months of treatment with ginkgo, the enzyme levels associated with liver fibrosis were significantly reduced, and all the patients showed signs of remission from their chronic infections. As a result of this study, it has been suggested that ginkgo extract is effective in arresting the development of liver scarring in chronic hepatitis.

Fibrosis
Tissue scarring associated with the healing of wounds when excessive collagen has been produced.

Ginkgo and Asthma

For centuries, Chinese herbalists put ginkgo seeds in soups and other foods as a treatment for asthma and bronchitis. Ginkgo is a strong inhibitor of platelet-activating factor and might, therefore, have some value in the prevention or treatment of asthma. Platelet-activating factor (PAF) is a problem because it increases allergic inflammation and may trigger bronchial constriction, making breathing difficult.

Scientists at Shanghai Medical University used the lung tissues of guinea pigs to test the effectiveness of ginkgo extract in reducing the effects of PAF and histamine, a compound in the body that causes the inflammatory response. The results, published in 2000, showed that ginkgo improved the pulmonary functions and reduced the tendency for the lung tissues to contract under the influence of PAF and histamine. The researchers concluded that ginkgo was a promising treatment for bronchial asthma.

In a second, recent study, researchers in Kuwait tested the effects of a ginkgo extract on the blood cells of people with asthma. They found that, in addition to suppressing PAF, ginkgo acted as an anti-inflammatory agent that suppressed immune system antigens involved in triggering asthma attacks. These results led them to conclude that ginkgo extract may offer a novel therapeutic treatment for asthma.

CHAPTER 8

How to Select and Use Ginkgo

This chapter will help you understand what to look for when selecting ginkgo extract, including which form to purchase, what to look for on a label, and how to interpret what you read.

As with most herbs, ginkgo biloba can be purchased in dried leaf form (for homemade tea or tinctures), in capsules of leaf powder, and as a standardized extract in prepared tinctures, capsules, or tablets.

Standardized Ginkgo

When choosing a brand of ginkgo, we recommend that you read the label carefully to make sure you are getting a standardized extract. Unlike synthetic drugs, which contain a single compound, herbs often have a variety of active ingredients. We need to have a way of *standardizing* the product; that is, have a consistent, measured amount of product per unit dose, whether it's a capsule, a tablet, or a tincture. To achieve this, one active ingredient is selected as the marker.

As previously noted, in the case of ginkgo, Dr. Willmar Schwabe of the large German phytomedicine company, Schwabe GmbH, developed an extract of ginkgo leaves known as EGb 761, the one principally used in clinical trials worldwide. It contains 24 percent flavone glycosides and 6 percent terpene lactones. Most types of ginkgo extract sold today are in this standardized form that he developed.

Standardized ginkgo extract is also available in drop form, with 9.6 mg of flavone glycosides and 2.4 mg of terpene lactones per dose.

How Standardized Ginkgo Extracts Are Made

Making the standardized ginkgo begins when the leaves of the male plant are harvested in late summer or early fall. Several factors affect the potency of the ginkgo plant, including where the ginkgo leaves are grown, the conditions under which they are harvested, and the harvesting method used. The quality of the active components can vary by as much as 300 percent, depending upon the location, time of year, and harvesting method. Growers monitor the quality of the leaves and harvest them when the concentrations of active ingredients are at optimal levels. The leaves are dried to remove three-fourths of the water and are then pressed to prevent fermentation. It takes fifty pounds of leaves to yield one pound of finished extract. The final processing takes two weeks and involves twenty-seven steps as the active ingredients get isolated and standardized to arrive at the final extract.

Since plants grow naturally, their content of active, or marker, ingredients will always vary. To account for these variations and ensure a standardized product, the manufacturer will adjust the proportions in an individual mixture.

Tablets, Capsules, or Tea?

Tablets and capsules are made from measured amounts of ginkgo extract and are the most common and convenient forms. Gelatin or vegetable-based capsules filled with ginkgo extract come in a variety of sizes and strengths, so read the labels to ensure the proper dose. Tablets are powdered ginkgo extract, compressed into a solid pill, often with a variety of filler ingredients.

Ginkgo Tinctures, Teas, and Infusions

The liquid tinctures, teas, and infusions are absorbed more rapidly, but, by the same token, they may not last as long in your system. Many herbalists recommend these forms because the act of tasting the herb allows us to begin the process of allowing it to heal us. Perhaps, too, signals get sent to the appropriate parts of the body in preparation for healing.

Tinctures are liquid extracts of the herb that are not generally standardized, but do keep the vital components intact, preserved in a liquid base. To make a tincture, an herb is extracted by soaking it in alcohol. Usually one part of the herbal material is mixed with five or ten parts of liquid by weight. In the case of ginkgo, an alcohol base is used. For those who prefer not to taste the alcohol, we recommend that you put the tincture in warm water or tea for a few minutes, and let the alcohol evaporate. This will eliminate the taste of alcohol.

Teas are prepared from the whole herb, which is purchased in dried form from specialty herb shops and made into teas, decoctions, or infusions.

Chinese medicine often uses a decoction, which is made by boiling the dried herbs in water to extract the medicine and then reducing the liquid to concentrate the tea.

An infusion is like tea, but weaker. It is made using the same method you use to make tea from tea leaves or tea bags. You pour boiling water over the herb, let it steep, strain the liquid (or remove the tea bag), and then drink the mixture.

Note: Ginkgo is a bitter astringent and ginkgo

teas and infusions have a slightly sour flavor. They may require a sweetener to make the taste more palatable.

Determining the Correct Dose of Ginkgo

Most clinical studies conducted with standardized, guaranteed-potency ginkgo biloba extract (containing 24 percent flavone glycosides and 6 percent terpene lactones) recommend taking 40 mg, three times a day, with meals, for a total of 120 mg per day.

Clinical studies on treating intermittent claudication (leg cramps), tinnitus (ringing in the ears), and vertigo generally use a higher dose of the standardized extract, 160–320 mg daily, divided into two or three equal doses.

Clinical studies on treating more serious conditions, such as Alzheimer's disease, cerebral insufficiency, memory loss and depression, have used doses of 120 mg of ginkgo, taken one to three times a day with meals.

These recommendations are guidelines only, based on research and clinical use. Each person is different. We recommend that you start at the low end, watch for a response, including unwanted effects, and adjust the dose accordingly. Don't be concerned about getting the exact recommended dosage. If you have the (most common) 60 mg extract, you will, of course, be taking multiples of 60 (60, 120, 180, etc.); a 40 mg extract will be in multiples of 40 (80, 120, 160, etc.).

Note: Since ginkgo is rapidly absorbed by the body and has a half-life of about three hours, ginkgo is most effective if taken three times a day, with meals. Again, if that is impractical, simply adjust this to your own lifestyle, and take your daily amount in two doses instead.

Improvements with ginkgo are often gradual and subtle. It may take from four to eight weeks before effects are noticed. In some cases, results may take up to six months to appear.

Many health practitioners recommend ginkgo as an ongoing supplement, especially for those over age fifty. In cases involving serious conditions, you may want to review your condition after thirty days to see if you need to lower or increase your dosage, depending upon the results and your reasons for taking ginkgo in the first place. Be sure to read the safety cautions in the next section, as well.

Checking Labels— Reading Between the Lines

Most herbal products, including ginkgo biloba, are regulated as dietary supplements. In 1994, the FDA's Dietary Supplement Health and Education Act (known as DSHEA) set new guidelines with regard to quality, labeling, packaging, and marketing of supplements. It also sparked a surge of interest in herbal products. DSHEA allows manufacturers to make "statements of nutritional support for conventional vitamins and minerals," but since herbs aren't nutritional in the conventional sense, DSHEA allows them to make only what they call "structure and function claims."

The label can explain how a vitamin or herb affects the structure or function of the body. However, it cannot make therapeutic or prevention claims, such as "Treats headaches fast," or "Cures the common cold." A ginkgo biloba label can say, "helps support memory and cognitive functions," but it can't say, "it helps treat the symptoms associated with Alzheimer's disease," although this is one of many reasons people choose to use it. That would mention the condition and the treatment, and would be considered a drug claim.

Companies use verbal acrobatics in labeling products, so as not to fall over this line. You the consumer suffer from this, of course. Ideally, we should be allowed to label all supplements so you would know exactly what condition the product was for, and its possible side effects. Since the labels give insufficient information, you should use good resources, such as this one, to educate yourself.

Know Your Maker— Quality Control Counts

The Federal Drug Administration (FDA) has requested that supplement manufacturers follow specific standards, or Good Manufacturing Practices (GMPs). These are standards regarding quality control, which are essential. The product must also contain exactly what the label claims, in terms of the active ingredients, and any fillers, or other components. Of course, even herbal products can contain possible contaminants, such as bacteria, molds, and pesticides, so the manufacturing facility should follow high standards of cleanliness and processing procedures.

Trade organizations for the industry, such as the American Herbal Products Association (AHPA) and the National Nutritional Food Association (NNFA), are helping to enforce these quality standards for herbal products among their members. Their members agree to adhere to these high standards, and continue to work together to maintain them. In general, we recommend buying herbal products from a recognized manufacturer.

It is vital for manufacturers of herbal products to be responsible and maintain their high standards. Otherwise, the poor standards practiced by a few companies will taint the entire industry, and threaten our freedom to have these products available to us.

Another organization, the Council for Responsible Nutrition, continues to play a leading role in ensuring good manufacturing processes. It has worked on a political and public level to both educate and help shape appropriate legislation to allow continued freedom in our use of supplements.

When choosing a brand of ginkgo, we recommend looking at the label to see if the manufacturer follows specific standards or Good Manufacturing Practices (GMPs). Also, look for companies that commit their own resources to researching their products.

In addition to manufacturing procedures, there is the issue of fair work practices and intellectual property rights. Many herbs are grown in underdeveloped countries that can easily be exploited by Westerners. Basically, the manufacturers should have a partnership-oriented, rather than domination-type relationship, respecting native rights, ensuring that the farming is sustainable and renewable, and that the financial rewards are fair. With herbs, we are dealing with a gift of nature, and it would be a poor practice to show anything but the highest respect for the land, the people, and the environment from which they come.

CHAPTER 9

GINKGO SAFETY AND CAUTIONS

Ginkgo is very safe. Extremely high doses have been given to animals without serious consequences. It has shown no toxicity to liver, kidneys, or new blood cell formation.

In all the clinical trials of ginkgo combined, involving a total of almost 10,000 people, the incidence of side effects produced by ginkgo extract was extremely small. Mainly there were a few cases of allergic skin reactions, dizziness, heartburn, nausea, and mild tension headaches. There were also a very few reports of an increased tendency for epistaxis—nosebleeds. This suggests that ginkgo's blood-thinning properties may increase the incidence of nosebleed in individuals prone to this problem, and they should check with their doctors prior to using ginkgo or combining it with other anticoagulant drugs.

Ginkgo and Pregnancy

Ginkgo appears to pose no danger to pregnant women or nursing mothers according to the current monograph of the German Commission E (equivalent to the United States Food and Drug Administration). However, this decision should be discussed with your health practitioner, as should any supplement or medication you take during pregnancy or while nursing.

Ginkgo and Overdose

While ginkgo is free of serious side effects, massive ginkgo overdoses have led to agitation, restlessness, and gastrointestinal distress.

Ginkgo and Drug Interactions

According to the Commission E Report, German medical authorities do not believe that ginkgo possesses many negative drug interactions. However, because of ginkgo's blood-thinning effects, due its ability to inhibit the platelet activation factor (PAF), authorities warn that it should not be combined with anticoagulants, or even aspirin.

For this same reason, we also recommend that you discontinue taking ginkgo at least two weeks prior to any surgical procedure.

Also, be sure to check with your physician before taking ginkgo if you are currently using any of the following medications:

1. Anticoagulants: Acetaminophen (Tylenol), aspirin, clopidogrel (Plavix), Dipyridamole (Persantine), Ticlopidine (Ticlid), and Warfarin (Coumadin).

2. MAO Inhibitors: Ginkgo may increase the effects of MAO inhibitors.

3. Thiazide diuretics: Ginkgo may increase blood pressure when used with thiazide diuretics.

Know When to Speak to Your Doctor

There are times when it's important to seek professional medical help—for example, in cases of deteriorating mental function, enlarged prostate, high blood pressure, liver ailments, or severe depression. All are potentially serious conditions and should be checked out before you embark on a self-treatment program with ginkgo.

In the best of all possible worlds, your doctor will be familiar with the use of ginkgo biloba, and will prescribe it as needed. We believe most doctors are motivated and curious to find the best, least harmful approaches to helping their patients. We therefore recommend that you take this book, or others like it, to your doctor to help inform him or her of the benefits of ginkgo biloba. Fortunately, those who seek complementary care tend to be the most likely to take responsibility for their own healing, and the least likely to expect the doctor to do or know it all. Sharing this knowledge can help you, your doctor, and his or her other patients.

CONCLUSION

Five thousand years ago, the legendary Chinese emperor Shen Nong, "wrested from Nature a knowledge of her opposing principles" to reveal the health-enhancing effects of ginkgo biloba, proclaiming that this gentle herb would allow one to follow the "Way of Long Life."

Today, Western researchers continue to add new and unexpected anti-aging and life-extending properties to an already impressive body of proven health benefits attributed to ginkgo.

First, acting as a potent antioxidant, ginkgo neutralizes free radicals to protect your cells and tissues, particularly those in your brain and your circulatory systems, the ones most prone to the ravages of aging. Second, ginkgo enhances the flow of blood in your arteries and capillaries to speed the delivery of life-giving nutrients and oxygen. And third, by inhibiting platelet activating factor (PAF), ginkgo keeps your blood from becoming sluggish, and prevents the formation of life-threatening blood clots.

Knowing about these essential properties helps you understand the wide array of important health benefits ginkgo offers you, including its ability to:

- Alleviate depression.

- Alleviate macular degeneration and improve visual acuity.

- Ameliorate intermittent claudication (leg pain due to poor blood flow when walking).

- Improve memory in both normal adults and those with Alzheimer's disease.

- Improve pulmonary function and relieve asthma.

- Improve sexual function and desire in both men and women.

- Inhibit platelet aggregation and the tendency for blood to clot abnormally.

- Reduce elevated blood pressure.

- Reduce or eliminate vertigo (dizziness and loss of stability).

- Relieve angina pectoris due to coronary artery disease (atherosclerosis).

- Relieve PMS symptoms, including edema.

- Relieve tinnitus (ringing in the ears).

In the short space of this book, we've seen how clinical research has proven the safety and effectiveness of this ancient herb, demonstrating how ginkgo protects and strengthens our bodies in a variety of ways that can help us live longer and healthier lives.

We wish to close with the reminder that ginkgo is an important natural resource. With ginkgo, as with all herbs, we must incorporate an appreciation for the gift that nature offers us and, even as we enjoy the bounty of the harvest, be sure to replant and renew.

Remember to honor your Mother, the earth, and walk lightly on her surface as you follow your "Way of Long Life."

SELECTED
REFERENCES

Bauer, U. 6-Month double-blind randomized clinical trial of Ginkgo biloba extract versus placebo in two parallel groups in patients suffering from peripheral arterial insufficiency. *Arzneimittelforsch,* 1984; 34:716–720.

Bruno, C, et al. Regeneration of motor nerves in bilobalide-treated rats. *Planta Medica,* 1993; 59:302–307.

Chatterjee, SS, et al. Studies on the mechanism of action of an extract of ginkgo biloba, a drug used for treatment of ischemic vascular diseases. *Archives of Pharmacology,* 1982; 320:R52.

Chung, KF, et al. Effect of a ginkgolide mixture (BN 52063) in antagonising skin and platelet responses to platelet activating factor in man. *Lancet,* 1987; 1:248–251.

Clostre, F. From the body to cell membranes: the different levels of action of Ginkgo biloba extract. *Presse-Medicale,* 1986; 15:1529–1538.

Coles, R. Trial of an extract of Ginkgo biloba (EGB) for tinnitus and hearing loss. *Clinical Otolaryngology and Allied Sciences,* 1988; 13:501–504.

De Long, Xie, Ning, et al. Ginkgo biloba composition, method to prepare the same and uses thereof, U.S. Patent, 6,030,621, Feb 29, 2000.

Doly, M, et al. Effect of Ginkgo biloba extract on the electrophysiology of the isolated diabetic rat retina. *Presse-Medicale*, 1986; 15:1480–1483.

Dubreuil, C. Comparative therapeutic trial of Ginkgo biloba extract and nicergoline in acute cochlear deafness. *Presse-Medicale*, 1986; 15:1559–1561.

Dumont, E, et al. Protection of polyunsaturated fatty acids against iron-dependent lipid peroxidation by a Ginkgo biloba extract (EGb 761). *Methods and Findings in Experimental and Clinical Pharmacology*, 1995; 17(2):83–88.

Emerit, I, et al. Radiation-induced clastogenic factors: anticlastogenic effect of Ginkgo biloba extract. *Free Radical Biology and Medicine*, 1995; 18:985–991.

Gebner, B, et al. Study of the long-term action of a Ginkgo biloba extract on vigilance and mental performance as determined by means of quantitative pharmaco-EEG and psychometric measurements. *Arzneimittelforsch*, 1985; 35:1459–1465.

Guillon, JM, et al. Effects of Ginkgo biloba extract on various in vitro and in vivo models of experimental myocardial ischaemia. *Presse-Medicale*, 1986; 15:1516–1519.

Haguenauer, JP, et al. Treatment of disturbances of equilibrium with Ginkgo biloba extract. A multicentre, double-blind, drug versus placebo study. *Presse-Medicale*, 1986; 15:1569–1572.

Huguet, F., and Tarrade, T. Alpha2-Adrenoceptor changes during cerebral ageing. The effect of ginkgo biloba extract. *Journal of Pharmacy and Pharmacology*, 1992; 44:24–27.

Haramaki, N, et al. Effects of natural antioxidant Ginkgo biloba extract (EGb 761) on myocardial ischemia-reperfusion injury. *Free Radical Biology and Medicine,* 1994; 16:789–794.

Hofferberth , B. Effect of ginkgo biloba extract on neurophysiological and psychometric measurement results in patients with cerebro-organic syndrome. A double-blind study versus placebo. *Arzneimittelforsch,* 1989; 39:918–922.

Hofferberth, B. The Efficacy of EGb 761 (Ginkgo biloba extract) in Patients with Senile Dementia of the Alzheimer Type, A Double-Blind, Placebo-Controlled Study on Different Levels of Investigation. *Human Psychopharmacology,* 1994; 9:215–222.

Holgers, K-M, et al. Ginkgo biloba extract for the treatment of tinnitus. *Audiology,* 1994; 33:85–92.

Jung, F, et al. Effect of Ginkgo biloba on fluidity of blood and peripheral microcirculation in volunteers. *Arzneimittelforsch,* 1990; 40:589–593.

Kanowski, S, et al. Proof of efficacy of the Ginkgo biloba special extract EGb 761 in outpatients suffering from mild to moderate primary degenerative dementia of the Alzheimer type or multi-infarct dementia. *Pharmacopsychiatry,* 1996; 29: 47–56.

Kleijnen, J, Knipschild, P. Ginkgo biloba for cerebral insufficiency. *British Journal of Clinical Pharmacology,* 1992; 34:352–358.

Kleijnen, J., and Knipschild, P. Ginkgo biloba, intermittent claudication and cerebral insufficiency. *Lancet,* 1992; 340:1136–1139.

Lagrue, G, et al. Idiopathic cyclic oedema. Role of capillary hyperpermeability and its correction by Ginkgo biloba extract. *Presse-Medicale,* 1986; 15: 1550–1553.

Le Bars, P., Katz, M., Berman, N., et al. A placebo-controlled, double-blind, randomized trial of an extract of ginkgo biloba for dementia. *JAMA*, 1997; 278(16):1327–1332.

Lebuisson, DA, Leroy, L, Rigal, G. Treatment of senile macular degeneration with Ginkgo biloba extract. A preliminary double-blind, drug versus placebo study. *Presse-Medicale*, 1986; 15: 1556–1558.

Meyer, B. A multicentre, randomized, double-blind drug versus placebo study of Ginkgo biloba extract in the treatment of tinnitus. *Presse-Medicale*, 1986; 15:1562–1564.

Mouren, X, et al. Study of the anti-ischemic action of EGB 761 in the treatment of peripheral arterial occlusive disease by TcPO2 determination. *Angiology*, 1994; 45:413–417.

Oberpichler, H, et al. Effects of Ginkgo biloba constituents related to protection against brain damage caused by hypoxia. *Pharmacological Research and Communications*, 1988; 20:349–368.

Otamiri, T, et al. Ginkgo biloba extract prevents mucosal damage associated with small-intestinal ischaemia. *Scandinavian Journal of Gastroenterology*, 1989; 24:666–670.

Pidoux, B. Effects of Ginkgo biloba extract on functional activity of the brain. Results of clinical and experimental studies. *Presse-Medicale*, 1986; 15: 1588–1591.

Pincemail, J, et al. Anti-radical properties of Ginkgo biloba extract. *Presse-Medicale*, 1986; 15:1475–1479.

Racagni, G, et al. Variations of neuromediators in cerebral ageing. Effects of Ginkgo biloba extract. *Presse-Medicale*, 1986; 15:1488–1490.

Rai, GS, et al. A double-blind, placebo-controlled study of Ginkgo biloba extract ("Tanakan") in elderly outpatients with mild to moderate memory impairment. *Current Medical Research and Opinion,* 1991; 12:350–355.

Rapin, JR, et al. Local cerebral glucose consumption. Effects of Ginkgo biloba extract. *Presse-Medicale,* 1986; 15:1494–1497.

Schaffler, K, et al. Double-blind study of the hypoxia-protective effect of a standardised Ginkgo bilobae preparation after repeated administration in healthy volunteers. *Arzneimittelforsch,* 1985; 35: 1283–1286.

Schubert, H, Halama, P. Depressive episode primarily unresponsive to therapy in elderly patients: efficacy of Ginkgo biloba extract (EGB 761) in combination with antidepressants. *Geriatr Forsch,* 1993; 3:45–53.

Shen, J-G, Zhou, D-Y. Efficiency of Ginkgo biloba extract (EGb 761) in antioxidant protection against myocardial ischemia and reperfusion injury. *Biochemical and Molecular Biology International,* 1995; 35:125–134.

Sikora, R, et al. Ginkgo biloba extract in the therapy of erectile dysfunction. *Journal of Urology,* 1989; 141:188A.

Spinnewyn, B, et al. Effects of Ginkgo biloba extract on a cerebral ischaemia model in gerbils. *Presse-Medicale,* 1986; 15:1511–1515.

Taillandier, J, et al. Ginkgo biloba extract in the treatment of cerebral disorders due to aging. *Presse-Medicale,* 1986; 15:1583–1587.

Tamborini, A, Taurelle, R. Value of standardized Ginkgo biloba extract (EGB 761) in the management of congestive symptoms of premenstrual syndrome. *International Journal of Gynecology and Obstetrics*, 1993; 88:447–457.

Taylor, JE. Binding of neuromediators to their receptors in rat brain. Effect of chronic administration of Ginkgo biloba extract. *Presse-Medicale*, 1986; 15:1491–1493.

Vesper, J, Hansgen, K-D. Efficacy of Ginkgo biloba in 90 outpatients with cerebral insufficiency caused by old age. Results of a placebo-controlled double-blind trial. *Phytomedicine*, 1994; 1:9–16.

Vorberg, G. Ginkgo biloba extract (GBE): a long-term study of chronic cerebral insufficiency in geriatric patients. *Clinical Trials Journal*, 1985; 22: 149–157.

Yan, L-J, et al. Ginkgo biloba extract (EGb 761) protects human low density lipoproteins against oxidative modification mediated by copper. *Biochemical and Biophysical Research Communications*, 1995; 212:360–366.

OTHER BOOKS
AND RESOURCES

Cass, Hyla. *Kava: Nature's Answer to Stress, Anxiety, and Insomnia.* Rocklin, CA: Prima Publishing, 1998.

Cass, Hyla. *St. John's Wort: Nature's Blues Buster.* Garden City Park, NY: Avery Publishing Group, 1998.

Cass, Hyla, and Patrick Holford. *Natural Highs: Supplements, Nutrition, and Mind/Body Techniques to Help You Feel Good All the Time.* New York, NY: Avery Penguin Putnam, 2002.

GreatLife Magazine
Consumer magazine with articles on vitamins, minerals, herbs, and foods.
Available for free at many health and natural food stores.

Let's Live Magazine
Consumer magazine with emphasis on the health benefits of vitamins, minerals, and herbs.
Customer service:
1-800-676-4333
P.O. Box 74908
Los Angeles, CA 90004
Subscriptions: 12 issues per year, $19.95 in the U.S.; $31.95 outside the U.S.

Physical Magazine
Magazine oriented to body builders and other serious athletes.

Customer service:
1-800-676-4333
P.O. Box 74908
Los Angeles, CA 90004
Subscriptions: 12 issues per year, $19.95 in the U.S.;
$31.95 outside the U.S.

The Nutrition Reporter™ newsletter
Monthly newsletter that summarizes recent medical research on vitamins, minerals, and herbs.

Customer service:
P.O. Box 30246
Tucson, AZ 85751-0246
e-mail: jack@thenutritionreporter.com
www.nutritionreporter.com
Subscriptions: $26 per year (12 issues) in the U.S.; $32
U.S. or $48 CNC for Canada; $38 for other countries

Ginkgo Biloba Extract: A Review
Alan R. Gaby, M.D.
www.thorne.com/altmedrev/fulltext/ginkgo1-4.html

Ohio State University Extension Fact Sheet
Human Nutrition and Food Management
1787 Neil Avenue, Columbus, OH 43210-1295
Herbals In Your Life
Herb and Drug Interactions
http://ohioline.osu.edu/hyg-fact/5000/5406.html

PubMed, National Library of Medicine
www.ncbi.nlm.nih.gov/entrez/query.fcgi

USDA, ARS, Genetic Resources Web Server
www.ars-grin.gov/duke/

U.S. Pharmacist
A Review of Herb-Drug Interactions: Documented and Theoretical
www.uspharmacist.com/NewLook/DisplayArticle.cfm?item_num=566

INDEX

Adenosine triphosphate
(ATP), 10
Age-related macular
degeneration, 46
Alzheimer's disease,
20–21
American Herbal
Products
Association, 70
Anticoagulents, 74
Antidepressants, 39
antioxidants, 9
ARMD. *See* Age-related
macular
degeneration.
Arrhythmia, 25–26
Asthma, 64
Atherosclerosis, 47

Balance disorders, 57
*Biochemistry and
Biology
International*, 27
Blood flow, 28–29
Blood pressure, high, 25
Blood vessels, 9
Brain, 15–22
aging and, 16
ginkgo biloba and,
15–22

Cataracts, 50–51
Cerebellum, 57
Cerebral hypoxia, 10
Cerebrovascular
insufficiency, 17
ginkgo biloba and,
17–19
Chernobyl disaster, 62
Chinese medicine, 6
Circulatory system,
23–24
Cochlea, 53–55
*Consumer's Guide to
Herbal Medicine*, 40
Council for Responsible
Nutrition, 71

Deafness, 53–55
Dementia, 19–20, 22
Depression, 61–62
Diabetes, 43–44
Diabetic retinopathy,
43–44
Dietary Supplement
Health and
Education Act, 69
Dioecious trees, 7–8
Doctor's advice, when to
seek, 74–75
Double-blind studies, 45

Dutch East India
    Company, 6

Edema, 60
Enzymes, 36
Erectile disfunction, 35
Eyes, 41–51

FDA. *See* Food and
    Drug
    Administration.
Fibrosis, 63
Flavone glycosides, 8
Fluid retention, 60–61
Food and Drug
    Administration, 37,
    69, 70, 73

GBE. *See* Ginkgo
    extract.
German Commission E,
    73, 74
German Ministry of
    Health Committee
    for Herbal
    Remedies, 62
Ginkgolide B, 10–11,
    27–28
Ginkgoaceae tree, 5
Ginkgo biloba, 5–13,
    15–22, 23–31, 33–40,
    41–51, 53–58, 59–64,
    65–71, 73–75, 77–78
    active compounds, 8
    as aphrodisiac, 40
    asthma and, 64
    balance and, 56–58
    bark, 7
    brain and, 15–22
    cataracts, and, 50–51

cautions, 73–75
cerebrovascular
    insufficiency and,
    17–19
chemistry of, 8
depression and,
    61–62
dizziness, 56–58
dosages, 68–69
drug interactions, 74
fluid retention and,
    60–61
fruit, 7
glaucoma and, 47–49
hearing disorders
    and, 53–58
heart and, 23–31
heart attacks and,
    26–27
heart tissues and,
    26–27
hepatitis B and, 63
high blood pressure
    and, 25
immune system and,
    50
imported into U.S.,
    7–8
infusions, 67
labeling, 69–70
leaves, 7, 26
macular degeneration
    and, 46
nuts, 7
PAF and, 10–11,
    27–28
premenstrual
    syndrome and,
    59–61
radiation and, 63

rice wine and, 7
safety and, 73–75
seeds, 7
selection of, 65–71
sex and, 33–40
standardization of, 65–66
sunburn and, 63
supplements, 66–71
tea, 7, 67
tinctures, 67
tinnitus, 55–56
use of, 65–71
UV-induced eye damage and, 49–50
vertigo and, 56–57
vision and, 41–51
Ginkgo extract, 13, 26, 66
Glaucoma, 47–49
    African Americans and, 48
Good Manufacturing Practices, 70, 71
Gymnosperm, 5

Han Dynasty, 6
Hearing disorders, 53–58
Heart and ginkgo biloba, 23–31
Heart attacks and ginkgo biloba, 26–27
Heart tissues and, 26–27
Hepatitis B, 63
Hypertension, 25

Immune system, 50
Impotence, 35

Intermittent claudication, 30–31

Journal of the American Geriatrics Society, 33
Journal of Urology, 38

Karch, Stephen, 40

Linnaeus, Carolus, 6

Macular degeneration, 46
Macular edema, 44
MAO inhibitors, 74
Materia Medica of Shen Nong, 6
Mayo Clinic, 33–34
Multi-infarct dementia, 22

National Ambulatory Medical Care Survey, 35
National Institutes of Health, 35
National Nutritional Food Association, 70
Neurotransmitters, 35
Nitric oxide, 35, 38, 40

Oxygen, 28–29

PAF. *See* Platelet-activating factor.
Pen T'sao Ching, 6
Placebo pill, 18
Platelet-activating

factor, 10–11, 24, 27–28, 45
Premenstrual syndrome, 59–61

Radiation, 62
Retina, 41–42
Retinal detachment, 44
Retinopathy, 43–46

Schwabe, Willmar, 8, 12, 24, 65
Schwabe GmbH, 12, 65
Selective serotonin reuptake inhibitors, 39–40
Sexual function, 33–40
   antidepressant-induced problems, 39–40
Shanghai Medical University, 64
Shen Nong Shi, Emperor, 6, 77
SSRIs. *See* Selective serotonin reuptake inhibitors.
Stroke, 9

Sunburn, 63

Terpene lactones, 10
Thiazide diuretics, 74
Tiberius Claudius, Emperor, 30
Tinnitus, 55–56

University of California-Berkeley, 27
UV-induced eye damage, 49–50

Vasodilator, 55,
Viagra, 36–38, 40
   side effects, 37
   women and, 37
Vision, 41–51

"Way of Long Life," 5, 77, 78
World Health Organization, 30

Yang, 7
Yin, 7
Yinhsing, 6

Printed in the USA
CPSIA information can be obtained
at www.ICGtesting.com
JSHW051957150824
68134JS00050B/82